the Lyme
Solution

the Lyme Solution

A 5-Part Plan to Fight the
Inflammatory Auto-immune Response
and Beat Lyme Disease

DARIN INGELS, ND, FAAEM

AVERY | AN IMPRINT OF PENGUIN RANDOM HOUSE | NEW YORK

AVERY

an imprint of Penguin Random House LLC
penguinrandomhouse.com

First trade paperback edition 2019
Copyright © 2018 by Darin Ingels, ND

Most Avery books are available at special quantity discounts for bulk purchase for
sales promotions, premiums, fund-raising, and educational needs. Special books
or book excerpts also can be created to fit specific needs. For details, write
SpecialMarkets@penguinrandomhouse.com.

ISBN 9780735216303 (hardcover)
ISBN 9780735216327 (ebook)
ISBN 9780735216310 (paperback)

Printed in the United States of America
1 3 5 7 9 10 8 6 4 2

Book design by Ellen Cipriano
Diagram on page 226 by Tanya Maiboroda

For all of my fellow Lymies.

May this book inspire you and help you to

find solutions to better health.

Contents

Foreword

It's likely that most people reading this book either know someone suffering from Lyme disease or have experienced this disease personally. For those who haven't, unfortunately, the odds are increasing that you will.

According to the Centers for Disease Control (CDC), Lyme disease is "the fastest growing vector-borne infectious disease in the United States," with more than three hundred thousand people per year infected annually. That is ten times more Americans than previously reported, according to the International Lyme and Associated Diseases Society (ILADS), an organization that promotes education on Lyme disease. It may surprise you to learn that no study in existence demonstrates that ten to twenty-one days of antibiotic therapy cures chronic Lyme disease. In other words, a rising vector-borne illness is now being treated with an unproven approach. It may work for some people, but many more fail to recover. And the disease persists. The end result is that millions of people are left struggling with a debilitating and chronic ailment on their own.

And what makes it worse is the persistent autoimmune problems that Lyme disease creates. In my *New York Times* bestselling books, *The Autoimmune Solution* and *The Thyroid Connection*, I talk about how microbes can trigger autoimmune disease, including Hashimoto's disease, rheumatoid arthritis, lupus, and multiple sclerosis. I have seen more and more people in my own practice whose autoimmune disease and chronic health problems are directly the result of Lyme disease. It is becoming increasingly clear that Lyme disease is more than just an infection that needs to be killed.

Enter *The Lyme Solution*. In this book, Dr. Ingels has recalibrated the lens through which we see and understand Lyme disease using the best twenty-first-century science and know-how. Currently, the health care system is making the poor trade-off in which ineffective attempts to kill off a complex bug (or, in reality, multiple bugs) wind up undermining the immune system—while rendering the bugs stronger. In contrast, *The Lyme Solution* plan strengthens and supports the immune system and thereby reduces symptoms, lessens infection, and ultimately defeats the invader. To any long-term Lyme sufferer I know, that will sound almost too good to be true. But it *is* true.

Dr. Ingels provides a true functional medicine approach to Lyme disease, not only looking at the infection itself, but also the myriad of other underlying problems that can weaken your immune system and makes Lyme disease worse. He clearly lays out a diet plan that can help improve your gut health and make you immune system stronger. Dr. Ingels shows you the importance of controlling your environment, avoiding toxic chemicals and mold, and living a healthier lifestyle, which can bring about positive changes in your overall health. Lyme disease is complicated and affects sufferers differently, but *The Lyme Solution* can help you start to heal and reclaim your health.

I've known Darin Ingels for several years and referred many of my own patients and friends—I myself have even sought out his advice—always with excellent results. To anyone who has followed the extraordinary health breakthroughs proffered by functional medicine, his approach makes total sense scientifically—and it also delivers practically. I know that from following the clinical results.

Make no mistake about it—*The Lyme Solution* is not a quick fix or a silver bullet. It is not as simple as swallowing a pill. It requires a commitment to your health. But most often, adjusting your diet and lifestyle, and following the clinically proven protocols to boost the immune system, will deliver what other approaches fail to: real results in managing your symptoms, restoring your health, and giving you back your life. And that is truly priceless!

Wishing you great health,
Amy Myers, MD

Part One

Introduction
to the
Lyme Solution

CHAPTER 1

Why Antibiotics Aren't Enough

Lyme disease can strike anyone anywhere. You don't need to live in a deer-ridden area of the East Coast of the United States. People from urban areas like New York City, Los Angeles, and Sydney, Australia, as well as arid places like Phoenix and Saudi Arabia, contract Lyme disease. It has been identified in more than eighty countries around the world.[1] Lyme has afflicted countless people in the public eye, including Avril Lavigne, Richard Gere, and George W. Bush. It's even gotten to the point that scientists have now identified the factors that determine a higher prevalence of ticks. Warmer weather increases the mice population, which transmits Lyme disease to deer.[2]

In addition to the growing number of Lyme cases, other insect-borne illnesses, such as Rocky Mountain spotted fever, dengue virus, malaria, and Zika virus are also on the rise. Some of these diseases are transmitted through a tick bite, like Lyme, but others are spread through the bites of mosquitoes, fleas, or flies. As I mentioned earlier, deer are not the only Lyme disease carriers. Other small animals, including mice, rats, rabbits, and squirrels, contribute to the spread of Lyme disease. Rising global temperatures will trend toward more insect-borne diseases in the coming years.[3]

The Discovery of Lyme Disease

No one knows exactly when Lyme disease started to emerge, but evidence suggests it has been around for thousands of years.[4] The oldest known person to have been exposed to *Borrelia* is "Ötzi the Iceman," a 5,300-year-old mummy found in the Austrian Alps.[5] Modern Lyme disease was rediscovered in 1975, when some children living near Lyme, Connecticut, started to experience symptoms that looked like juvenile rheumatoid arthritis, a rare condition. Because far more children were affected than the national average, their illness began to be referred to as "Lyme arthritis." Several adults in the area had similar symptoms. When a rheumatologist at Yale University began to treat some of them with antibiotics, many improved, suggesting some type of bacteria had caused the arthritis.[6]

But the true culprit of Lyme disease had yet to be identified. In the early 1980s, tick samples were sent to Dr. Willy Burgdorfer, a microbiologist and expert in Rocky Mountain spotted fever, to figure out what was causing this mysterious inflammatory infection. Although he was looking for a different infection, he noticed spirochetes—flexible, spiral-shaped bacteria—in many of the ticks he had tested. When he tested people with Lyme disease, he found they had the identical bacteria. Burgdorfer published his research in 1984, making the link between this newly discovered spirochete and Lyme disease. The organism was aptly named *Borrelia burgdorferi* in honor of his finding. Once scientists started to realize that *Borrelia* caused more than just arthritis, it was renamed *Lyme disease*.

Lyme disease is complicated for many reasons that this book will reveal. For one thing, current testing is woefully inadequate. The Lyme organism itself morphs to hide from the immune system. Nor is there any one treatment for everyone with Lyme disease. Doctors and other health-care providers lack Lyme awareness, especially in areas of the world where it is not considered common. All of these factors make it difficult to get an accurate diagnosis and early and proper treatment.

Many lives and careers have been ruined by Lyme disease. Suicide rates are higher among people with chronic Lyme. Some people are wiped out financially. And most health insurance companies will cover only twenty-eight days or so of antibiotic treatment. As a physician friend of mine remarked, "That may be enough to get rid of your bull's-eye rash, but it's often not enough to get rid of the Lyme." With Lyme now epidemic, the health-care system has a long way to go. Long-range approaches to a complex and volatile ailment like Lyme are not its strong suit.

I wrote *The Lyme Solution* to be a straightforward, easy-to-read guide on how people with Lyme disease can take control of their own health and make use of new, innovative treatments that have not been widely offered before. My new and unique understanding about the interaction between your immune system and the Lyme bug will upgrade your ability to treat and recover from Lyme disease and become Lyme-free at last.

I am a naturopathic physician with practices in both Connecticut and California, a board member of the American Association of Naturopathic Physicians, and the author of two books and numerous articles. I know firsthand what it's like for patients to experience an odd variety of apparently unrelated symptoms—symptoms that have other doctors scratching their heads. I know because I personally struggled with Lyme disease—and cured myself. And out of that struggle to treat my own Lyme, I developed a radical and highly effective new treatment approach that has helped thousands of others.

Highly regarded integrative and functional medical doctors refer their patients to me. And often they come for themselves. They know that I have the practical tools and knowledge to address this rising epidemic. That's why I have written *The Lyme Solution*: to offer my revolutionary new view of this disease, a view that finally makes it possible to prevent and treat a puzzling ailment that so often leaves both patients and their doctors in what I call the "Lyme quagmire"—exhausted, overwhelmed, feeling terrible, and wandering desperately from treatment to treatment without achieving complete and long-term recovery. That can and must stop!

But be prepared: my approach to treating and beating Lyme is nothing like the one most doctors use to treat people with Lyme disease. The irony of conventional Lyme treatment is that the very protocol doctors routinely offer exacerbates Lyme symptoms and undermines your chance of long-term recovery. No one can treat Lyme if their basic understanding of it is wrong.

Discarding the all-too-common misunderstandings about this dreadful disease will save you from wasting your precious time and health on protocols that actually worsen the outcome, only to find yourself back at square one.

The Immune-Boosting Plan

The Immune-Boosting Plan featured in this book will help you kill the infection naturally and safely, improve your nutrition, and boost your immune system. I also offer recommendations to control the nagging symptoms that have kept you from feeling well. For some of the therapies or tests I cover, you might need to consult with your doctor or health-care provider. By reading *The Lyme Solution*, you will know what to ask them so that you can get the best test or treatment.

In this chapter, you will learn why the most widely used treatment—antibiotics—is not always effective and can even be counterproductive. I will also introduce you to autoimmune dysfunction and reveal what occurs in the body during an autoimmune response. In Chapter 2, I address the complex and controversial issue of diagnosing Lyme disease. I will cover in detail the problems and pitfalls with each of the currently available tests. With my clear assessment of all these tests, you will bypass unnecessary confusion to understand why these tests are so often inadequate and miss many people with Lyme disease. With that knowledge, you can use some of them to your advantage. You can also take the Lyme Disease Symptom Questionnaire (page 42) to figure out whether you are likely to have Lyme disease.

Part Two, Chapters 3 through 7, takes you through the five major steps of the Immune-Boosting Plan. You will customize this plan to your own needs, depending on whether you currently are:

- reducing your risk of Lyme if you reside in a Lyme-saturated region,
- suspicious that you may have recently been bitten by a tick,
- treating acute Lyme in the wake of a recent tick bite or rash, or
- experiencing chronic Lyme.

In Chapter 3, you begin the plan with gut- and immune-restoring protocols. I'll also cover what contributes to autoimmunity, explaining why gut health is so important to bringing the immune response back into balance.

Chapter 4 introduces the Immune-Boosting Diet and shows how and why following the diet will recalibrate your health. The food lists, menu plans, and delicious recipes (found at the end of the book) will help you achieve the critical goal of alkalinizing your body so that each cell is working the way it should. You will learn why alkalinity is paramount for Lyme recovery and master which foods to eat and which to avoid. (Recipes for the Immune-Boosting Diet begin on page 273.)

In Chapter 5, I'll help you target active infection in a way that doesn't disrupt your gut flora or undermine your immune system. My herbal protocols will reduce your body's load of Lyme without making you feel sick or nauseated. I will offer you several potent herbal protocols and help you determine which one(s) are likely best for you. Life is different when you have a clear strategy for managing and recovering from Lyme.

In Chapter 6 you will learn why cleaning up your home or work environment is a simple way to improve your health. By avoiding toxic cleaners, pesticides, air fresheners, and other household chemicals, you remove the toxic burden that suppresses your immune system and makes you sick. Mold in your home exacerbates many Lyme symptoms. This chapter will show you how to find out if you might have mold, how to test for it, and how to get rid of it.

Chapter 7 focuses on sleep, exercise, and stress reduction—crucial steps in the road to recovery. Most of your tissue repair occurs when you sleep. Your nervous system winds down and restores your energy. That's why it's essential that people with Lyme disease learn ways to get deep, restorative sleep. Poor circulation is common with Lyme disease and can lead to reduced levels of oxygen and nutrients. In this chapter, you will start a gentle and doable exercise plan that can help get your blood moving again. Finally, managing your stress will also help you feel better and retain a healthier frame of mind. This chapter will show you ways to reduce your stress.

Part Three focuses more sharply on chronic Lyme. In Chapter 8 you'll learn about more-advanced protocols that you can use to target specific symptoms. These include novel ways of improving your immune system, such as sublingual or low-dose immunotherapy. For these, you will need to work with a health-care provider, as these need to be medically managed. This chapter will also share other procedures and medications that have helped many people with Lyme disease.

Finally, in Chapter 9, *The Lyme Solution* will review what you should do if, after going through the Immune-Boosting Plan, you are still struggling. It explains why it's often beneficial to cycle back through the plan once you are familiar with it. In some cases, there may be other reasons why you are not getting better. This book will discuss other conditions that people with Lyme confront that can be treated in other ways. Lab tests will help you and your doctor pinpoint other related health concerns to address. This will help you and your doctor come up with the next steps in your journey to feeling well again.

The World of Lyme Disease

Lyme disease has become the fastest-growing insect-borne infectious disease in the United States, Europe, and Asia.[7] For people who work and play outdoors, checking for deer ticks will eventually become as routine as brushing your teeth. More than 300,000 people each year in the United States and 65,000 people in Europe are affected by this epidemic—and for reasons I'll make clear, many more cases go unreported or are undiagnosed.[8]

Although a bull's-eye rash and flu-like symptoms are the classic early signs of Lyme, many people never experience either. Some people get vague symptoms (or none at all) and may harbor the infection for years without knowing it. Hundreds of thousands of people have the typical symptoms of Lyme without even knowing that they have the disease—until long after it has deeply entrenched itself into their bodies. Many more seek out medical help for chronic cases of Lyme only to find that medicine has little to offer. Often they are misdiagnosed or improperly treated. In many cases, their concerns are dismissed. From the moment people first notice a tick bite, all the way through to the time when they get a Lyme diagnosis, people with Lyme disease need the right answers. And they need them right away. Why? Because the way you treat Lyme once it's contracted will make a huge difference in whether you end up living Lyme-free.

Yet confirming that you have Lyme can itself be a major hurdle. Because it hides in the body and mimics other diseases, Lyme is notoriously hard to diagnose. On top of that, there is no real medical consensus on Lyme diagnosis or treatment. It's quite common for well-intentioned doctors to prescribe antibiotics for months to years, often with no end in sight. Although this is one bug you really want to try to kill as quickly as possible, antibiotic treatment all too often undermines your best long-term defense against it.

In contrast to the long-term use of antibiotics, most people use my program for just three to six months. Both quicker and more effective than other treatments, it has helped thousands of people with Lyme disease find relief. This book is different from any other book on Lyme disease because I focus not just on the Lyme infection itself, but on the chronic, inflammatory autoimmune response that Lyme triggers. I treat Lyme disease in the way that I have discovered works best—as an inflammatory autoimmune response by a system that has been on high alert for too long. That is what has to be addressed—and round after round of antibiotic cocktails will only make it harder to do that. My Immune-Boosting Plan will help you dial down the inflammation, calm the triggered reactions, support your immune system, and recover your health.

The goal of this book is to give you a road map to navigate your

Lyme disease and become your own best advocate for your health. You can safely follow nearly all of my Immune-Boosting Plan on your own. I will also reveal how to develop a partnership with a health-care provider who can get you the lab tests or therapies that require medical supervision or a prescription. My approach shifts the focus from killing Lyme bacteria to addressing the autoimmune condition triggered by the Lyme. Your body can fight Lyme disease, but you have to know how to use and strengthen your immune system.

In early Lyme disease, antibiotic therapy may kill the spirochetes before your immune system responds. But in chronic Lyme disease, the activation of your immune system itself is causing the symptoms.

In any autoimmune condition, your body starts to attack its own tissues, mistakenly believing that they are the invading organism it is supposed to defeat. That's why instead of prescribing heavy rounds of antibiotics, I start from the premise that the later-stage symptoms of Lyme disease are due not to the infection itself but to your body attacking its own healthy tissues. This opens the way to using effective diet modifications and therapies to support the immune system, eliminate the infections, and lessen the autoimmune reactivity.

Overcoming Lyme disease can be challenging, but it is possible. Taking the steps outlined in this book is the best place to start. There is power in knowledge. I look forward to the day when you too are Lyme-free.

The Acute and Chronic Stages of Lyme Disease

If you value your health and spend time outdoors, you must familiarize yourself with—and protect yourself from—Lyme. When one little bite can lead to a host of minor and major debilitating symptoms, it's essential to learn how to check for ticks and know exactly what to do if you find them. With or without a visible bite, it's urgent that people learn to identify Lyme's characteristic symptoms, so that they can begin treatment as soon as possible—before the disease progresses.

Instant action is a necessity because, if left untreated, early Lyme can morph into chronic Lyme disease. An acute case of Lyme disease consists of symptoms that develop within days or weeks of a tick bite and may be treated relatively easy at the outset. A chronic case occurs when Lyme makes its way deep into your system and keeps recurring, possibly with periods of remission. Both types of Lyme are misunderstood.

The early acute phase of Lyme disease generally occurs from three to thirty days after a tick bite.

Signs and Symptoms of Early Acute Lyme Disease

- Fever
- Chills
- Pounding, throbbing headache
- Persistent noticeable fatigue
- Numbness and tingling
- Muscle and joint aches
- Swollen lymph nodes
- Facial or Bell's palsy (loss of muscle tone, or drooping on one or both sides of the face)
- Erythema migrans (EM) rash (bull's-eye rash)

The most well-known and characteristic symptom of the acute phase is the EM or bull's-eye rash. It begins at the site of a tick bite, expanding until it reaches up to twelve inches or more across. Rarely itchy or painful, this rash sometimes clears as it enlarges, so that it resembles a target or bull's-eye.

If you were lucky enough to catch your Lyme disease early, you got rid of the infection and felt fine afterward. If not, it's likely that you struggled. You may have made multiple visits to numerous doctors over months, maybe years, with no definitive answers. Your declining health deeply affects your life. You may have been diagnosed with chronic fatigue syndrome, fibromyalgia, restless legs syndrome, depression, neuropathy, multiple sclerosis, or some other illness that seems vague and has no real known cause. If you're reading this book, my guess is that you—or perhaps a loved one who has undergone this puzzling journey—continue to suffer.

If not treated early (or correctly), Lyme may become chronic. Here,

Symptoms of Chronic Lyme Disease

- Severe headaches
- Neck stiffness
- Persistent fatigue and exhaustion
- Additional EM rashes or other skin rashes around the body
- Arthritis with severe joint pain and swelling, especially in the knees and other large joints
- Pain in tendons, muscles, joints, and bones, intermittently
- "Wandering" pains from location to location
- Irregular heartbeat (Lyme carditis) or heart palpitations
- Dizziness or shortness of breath
- Inflammation of the brain and spinal cord
- Nerve pain
- Shooting pains, numbness, tingling, or burning sensations in the hands or feet
- Problems with short-term memory

too, there is no definitive profile. Thousands of people with long-term Lyme disease experience an extensive menu of now-you-feel-it-now-you-don't complaints. Typically, people with chronic Lyme disease report having at least three out of the many possible symptoms.

Customary approaches to Lyme disease often miss the mark. Conventional doctors view Lyme as an infection to stamp out with antibiotics. But unless antibiotics are administered within seventy-two hours of a deer tick bite, they have a poor track record.[9]

Once Lyme disease progresses to the chronic stage, many conventional doctors double down on this same approach, administering heavy, long-term doses of antibiotic cocktails that they hope will knock out the bacteria in all of its various disguises. But long-term treatment with antibiotics doesn't fare much better. When symptoms don't abate, some doctors will keep their patients on high doses of these drugs for a month or longer. By then, the immune system may be too weakened from antibiotics to fight off the next round of belligerent Lyme. Overall, up to two thirds of people with Lyme disease will fail conventional antibiotic therapy.[10]

Sometimes this mode of treatment will temporarily cause symptoms to abate, misleading people into thinking they are cured—when they aren't. Later, when they least expect it, the elusive or dormant Lyme spirochetes easily reactivate themselves, producing a sudden relapse or unexpected symptoms.

PETER'S STORY

Peter, the nine-year-old son of friends, had come to my practice for seasonal allergies and general immune support. One day his mother called to say he had started jerking his head and blinking his eyes. Tests showed he had elevated antibodies to strep. I knew of a condition triggered by exposure to strep called PANS (pediatric acute-onset neuropsychiatric syndrome) that produces tics, obsessive-compulsive disorder (OCD), anxiety, and other neurological problems. While he was undergoing treatment for strep, his symptoms mildly improved, but did not completely go away.

At one of our follow-up appointments, Peter's mother mentioned that he had had Lyme disease at age four but was treated with antibiotics and had no further symptoms. When I ran a blood test for Lyme disease, it came back positive.

I started Peter on the Modified Cowden Protocol (featured in Chapter 5), which helps the body rid itself of Lyme and other infections. I often use this protocol with children under age eight, as well as adults who don't like swallowing capsules. The liquid tinctures of Samento, Banderol, and Cumanda helped to treat Peter's Lyme disease. I also gave him low-dose immunotherapy Lyme 12C (discussed in Chapter 8). Within days of starting his treatment, his symptoms completely went away. After almost ten months, the tics have still not returned.

As you can see from Peter's story, undiagnosed chronic Lyme can arise later to produce unexpected symptoms. It can also imitate, contribute to, and often worsen many other serious illnesses. Because of overlapping symptoms, it is often mistaken for:

Chronic fatigue syndrome
Fibromyalgia
Rheumatoid arthritis
Multiple sclerosis
Parkinson's disease
Amyotrophic lateral sclerosis (ALS)
and many other chronic health conditions

Ironically, treating Lyme may contribute to recovery from these other conditions. But because of inadequate medical understanding of both Lyme and these other disorders, the result is all too often confusion.

Deceiving Your Immune System

One of the greatest challenges in treating Lyme successfully is that your body doesn't detect the Lyme bug. In sharp contrast to other common infections, the Lyme bacteria is surprisingly adept at concealing itself from your immune system. In fact, the moment a tick pierces your skin, it coats the Lyme bacteria with its saliva. As Lyme hides within that protective coating, it may take weeks before your immune system even recognizes its opponent and starts producing antibodies to fight it off. This explains why tests for Lyme given too soon after a bite so often come up negative—an extremely common result that has long baffled both people with Lyme disease and their doctors.

The Lyme bacteria also has a unique shape. Known as a spirochete because of its flagella (slender, threadlike appendages) and its long, spiral form, the Lyme bug can travel easily through the tissues of your body, twisting and turning as it elongates. It is one of the few bacteria that can change its shape to hide from your immune system or become more resistant to antibiotics.[11] The human body contains over 100 trillion bacteria, each uniquely different. *Borrelia*—the scientific name for Lyme bacteria—is the most clever and adaptable of them all.

The Lyme spirochete is in the same family as other spirochetes, such as *Treponema pallidum* (the bacterium that causes syphilis) and *Leptospira interrogans* (a cause of meningitis). Famously tough to diagnose, diseases caused by spirochetes are easily mistaken for other ill-nesses. And because they hide so successfully, spirochete diseases can invade your tissues without your knowledge and cause problems years, even decades, after that first infection. This produces the sudden re-lapses that many people with chronic Lyme disease report.

The shape-shifting Lyme bacteria can send your immune system on a wild-goose chase. Each time the versatile spirochete changes, the immune system has to devise a different way to defeat it. But by the time the immune system does so, the devilish Lyme bacteria has morphed yet again. In this back-and-forth process of evading your im-mune system, the shape-shifter has ample time to establish itself inside you. The result? The Lyme has a solid foothold, while the various an-tibodies launched against it trigger the inflammation and discomfort so many endure.

The Lyme spirochete can also go completely dormant inside the body—a little like rolling over and playing dead. In that condition, it is less vulnerable to antibody attack and continues to persist. Lyme has even developed the uncanny knack of hiding itself inside scar tissue, which is out of the immune system's reach. A 2011 study at the Univer-sity of California uncovered an even more remarkable strategy: Lyme spirochetes can hide in your lymph nodes, in the immune system itself—behind enemy lines, so to speak.[12]

People with Lyme disease are likely to be the most symptomatic when the *Borrelia* spirochetes are active and moving throughout the body. But even then, when antibiotics have the best chance of killing Lyme, laboratory studies have shown that *Borrelia* can literally coil it-self into a ball, known as a "round body," so that your immune system is unable to detect and eradicate it.[13] While an average sinus infection might last a week or so, Lyme can remain in the body for months and years. These round-body forms have been found even in the spinal fluid of people with Lyme disease, where they affect the central nervous system. This may also explain why treating Lyme disease of the brain, which causes headaches, dizziness, memory problems, neuropathy, poor balance, and difficulty walking, is so problematic.[14]

Lyme Disease and Other Uninvited Guests

To further complicate matters, when you get a tick bite, you may also get other infections. Many ticks that carry Lyme disease also carry a host of other infections that can be transmitted through the same bite and produce many of the same symptoms as Lyme disease. That's why, when you get tested for Lyme (see Chapter 2), it is a good idea to test for all of these co-infections at the same time so that you and your doctor know what you are treating. Some of the other illnesses that look like Lyme disease include *Bartonella*, *Babesia*, *Anaplasma*, *Ehrlichia*, *Rickettsia*, *Mycoplasma*, Powassan virus, Colorado tick fever, tularemia, and relapsing tick fever.

Every year, researchers discover more and more new bacteria and viruses transmitted through tick bites. At first, researchers thought it was only a handful of bugs, but in fact there are potentially *hundreds* of different microbes that can infect humans and make us sick. Some of the more common co-infections are listed in Appendix A (page 329). If you have Lyme-like symptoms and all your tests come up negative, I recommend talking with your doctor to test for other bugs that might be making you ill.

Borrelia and Its Transmission

There are more than a hundred different species of *Borrelia* in the United States and more than three hundred worldwide. The most common, *Borrelia burgdorferi*, with fifteen subspecies, causes most of the cases of Lyme disease in the United States.[15] In addition to *Borrelia burgdorferi*, *Borrelia garinii*, *Borrelia afzelii*, and *Borrelia miyamotoi* are common species responsible for Lyme disease in the United States and Europe.[16] Even among different strains of *Borrelia burgdorferi*, there are genetic differences between the Lyme bacteria found in the United States and those found in Europe.[17] This suggests an incredibly complex organism that can adapt to different environments easily to maintain its survival.

The deer ticks that transmit the *Borrelia* organism are primarily from the *Ixodes* (pronounced "IK-so-deez") family. There are several types of *Ixodes* ticks. In the United States, *Ixodes scapularis* is the dominant Lyme-spreading tick on the East Coast, while *Ixodes pacificus* is responsible for most Lyme disease on the West Coast. You can see pictures of them at lymediseaseassociation.org/about-lyme/tick-vectors/photos.

While the name *deer tick* implies that people are exposed in areas infested with deer, this is not always true. The *Borrelia* themselves come mostly from small animals like mice or birds. The deer are merely transient hosts. In other words, you don't need to live in a wooded area with lots of deer to get Lyme disease.

Ticks go through a life cycle from egg to adult. They are most dangerous to humans at their intermediate nymph stage. Because the nymphs are so small, they are almost undetectable to the human eye. Nor can you feel a tick bite, unlike a mosquito bite or bee sting. A nymph is about the size of a pinhead, only 1 to 2 millimeters long. If one gets on your skin, you are unlikely to see it. Ticks also like to go to areas of your body that are dark and warm, such as your groin, your armpit, in your hair, or on the back of your knee. Since these are not parts of your body that you can see standing in front of a mirror, it's easy to miss a tick that has attached to your skin.

According to the Centers for Disease Control and Prevention (CDC), ticks must be attached to your skin for thirty-six to forty-eight hours before they can transmit Lyme to your blood.[18] However, one study found that some ticks can transmit Lyme disease within sixteen hours of attachment.[19] Newer research has shown that Lyme can be transmitted in less than twelve hours of tick attachment and other coinfections can be transmitted in under an hour. So to reduce your risk of infection, you should remove a tick as quickly as possible if you see one on you. Please see "How to Remove a Tick" on page 45. The sooner it's removed once it attaches, the less likely you are to get Lyme disease.

New evidence has shown that a pregnant mother with Lyme disease can transmit the infection to her child. Studies show that mothers with Lyme disease have a higher rate of complications at birth and more children born with birth defects.[20] This underlines the importance of doing comprehensive testing for all tick-borne illnesses in pregnant women who are suspected of having Lyme disease.

If a tick does infect you, there are no early warning signs. Although most people will start to feel sick within a few days of the bite, it can take up to thirty days or more after exposure before you become symptomatic. But because the symptoms are often vague, it can take months and sometimes years for many people to get a diagnosis. Chapter 2 discusses this issue at length.

Antibiotic Therapy: The Good, the Bad, and the Ugly

Most of my colleagues who treat Lyme disease aim to kill the organism as quickly as possible, using whatever combination of antibiotics it takes. This makes perfect sense, theoretically. But they fail to recognize that Lyme disease isn't just an infection but a complex medical problem that causes immune dysfunction, inflammation, circulation problems, and hormone imbalances. So if you target only one aspect of the problem, you're not getting to the root of the entire illness. The goal is to treat *you*.

I am not opposed to using antibiotics to treat Lyme disease when the person is a good candidate. When I initially had Lyme disease, I took antibiotics and within a few days of treatment felt much better. So antibiotics certainly are appropriate for the right person at the right time. The conventional medical treatment for Lyme disease is to take antibiotics for up to three weeks after diagnosis. This has been the recommendation of most government, medical, and public health organizations in the United States for almost forty years. (See Appendix B, page 332, for the CDC's detailed guidelines for treatment of Lyme disease.) While mainstream infectious-disease doctors do not generally deviate from the CDC recommendations, others feel that the standard twenty-one days of antibiotic therapy are not enough to defeat Lyme disease. Many of these doctors will use longer courses of antibiotics, both oral and intravenous, for weeks, months, or even years. Using up to three or four antibiotics at once is now common.

The good news is that some people get Lyme disease, take the recommended antibiotics, and never seem to have any further problems. Their symptoms go away. According to the CDC, antibiotics work most of the time, and only a small percentage of patients go on to develop chronic problems after their tick bite. Unfortunately, this is a skewed finding, because it refers primarily to people with known, acute Lyme disease who get early treatment. Yes, in this narrow range of cases antibiotics do seem to be an effective treatment. My guess is that if you are reading this book, the twenty-one days of doxycycline you took did not cure your Lyme disease.

LILY'S STORY

Lily had always been a healthy woman who enjoyed mountain biking, camping, and skiing with her husband. A successful attorney with two children, she is conscientious about her and her family's diet. But starting a few months ago, she began to feel pain in her joints and muscles when she got up in the morning. Her energy was low. At work, she forgot important details and could not complete important tasks on time.

When her primary doctor ran a few standard blood tests, they all came back negative. He recommended that she work on getting more rest and on managing her stress. But Lily's fatigue worsened to the point where she could barely get out of bed. Even the ibuprofen didn't help her painful joints, which now hurt all day. Irritable at home, she began to snap at her kids and husband for no reason, hating herself for it afterward. Her doctor ran more blood tests, including several for autoimmune and Lyme disease, but they, too, all came back negative. He referred her to a rheumatologist.

When the tests the rheumatologist did came back negative, he offered her medication to treat the pain. It didn't help. Lily began experiencing more stomach problems and was referred to a gastroenterologist, who did an endoscopy—but it, too, came back negative. The gastroenterologist prescribed more medication for her stomach complaints. Lily then started having daily headaches with numbness in her feet. Her doctor sent her to a neurologist, who did a computerized tomography (CT) scan of her brain and other neurological tests. All were normal. The doctors told her they could not find anything wrong with her.

A doctor Lily's friend recommended suspected she had Lyme disease. Although a previous Lyme test was negative, this doctor ran a more comprehensive one, which showed that she had both Lyme disease and another bacterial infection transmitted through a tick bite. Finally, after several months, Lily had found an answer! As soon as the doctor started her on combination antibiotics, her symptoms improved. She was overjoyed—until after a few weeks she experienced stomach pain and diarrhea.

Her doctor changed her treatment, using different antibiotics, which stopped the stomach pain and diarrhea, but then her symptoms flared again. Her joints were more painful. Her energy was worse. The doctor told her this was a normal die-off reaction that would subside within a matter of days, but it didn't. Instead, it went on for weeks without improvement. For the next few months, Lily's doctor kept changing her antibiotics, trying to find the combination that would get her over the hump. Instead, Lily developed a lot of side effects from the medication. Discouraged, unsure what to do next, she now had a real dilemma: she had Lyme disease and antibiotics weren't working.

The Downside to Antibiotics

Like Lily, many people come to my clinic after antibiotic treatment has failed to resolve their Lyme disease. Although they often have lost hope, I am able to reassure them that there are better treatment options. As I've mentioned, the most common conventional treatment works in some cases, and in others it makes the disease harder to cure. Why? Because long-term use of antibiotics kills off a large portion of your normal gut bacteria, which maintains the health of your immune system as well as fighting infection. The destruction of friendly bacteria creates a disrupted gut ecology, making your immune system less efficient in getting rid of infections.[21] Long-term antibiotics can also lead to kidney and liver damage and many other harmful side effects.

Having seen thousands of people with Lyme disease, I've witnessed the damaging effects of antibiotics—chronic abdominal pain, diarrhea, nausea, vomiting, headaches, and worsening of their fatigue and insomnia—on people who have been treated with them for months to years. According to the CDC, up to 20 percent of people with acute Lyme disease will fail antibiotic therapy and go on to develop post-treatment Lyme disease syndrome, with persistent fatigue, joint pain, muscle aches, and neurological problems.[22] New research on Lyme disease shows that some of the *Borrelia* organisms have become resistant to often-used antibiotics in treating Lyme disease and are called *persister* cells. These persister bacteria have developed clever ways of altering hundreds of their genes, making them well suited to survive antibiotics.[23] The persister bacteria seem to survive because they grow at a slower rate than other *Borrelia* organisms, giving the antibiotics less time to eradicate the infection.[24] Some new research is finding that certain antibiotics are better than others at eliminating persister bacteria.[25] However, many of these drugs, including dapsone and clofazimine (old drugs to treat leprosy), are potentially toxic and have many side effects.

Lyme Bacteria Replicate Slowly

Many antibiotics do not directly kill bacteria but work mainly by stopping them from reproducing. There is a window of opportunity when the bacterial cells are dividing during which the antibiotics are most effective. But Lyme bacteria replicate at a much slower rate than other bacteria. Most bacteria in your body reproduce exponentially every twenty minutes, which is pretty fast. However, the Lyme spirochete replicates every one to sixteen days.[26]

So instead of the typical ten to fourteen days of antibiotics to treat a sinus infection, for Lyme you would need to keep antibiotics in your system for up to eighteen months to have the same effect! That can harm you as much as it harms Lyme bugs.

There are millions of beneficial bacteria in your gut and elsewhere in and on your body. Since antibiotics can't distinguish between the good and bad bacteria, they target them all. And since friendly bacteria replicate rapidly, they are more susceptible to the antibiotics' damaging effects. Destroying the good ones leaves the field open to the baddies. Unopposed, they populate the digestive tract, causing gut and immune problems.

The Evidence Against Long-Term Antibiotic Use

A 2016 study conducted in Europe gave 280 people with Lyme disease two weeks of intravenous antibiotics followed by twelve weeks of doxycycline, clarithromycin plus hydroxychloroquine, or placebo. At the end of the trial, there was no difference between the treatment groups and the placebo group in quality of life or physical symptoms.[27] A test-tube study found that doxycycline and cefuroxime (Ceftin), two drugs commonly used to treat Lyme, were unable to kill persistent *Borrelia burgdorferi*.[28] Another study found that people with post-treatment Lyme disease of the brain and many other conditions had mild cognitive improvement while on intravenous ceftriaxone, but this benefit was lost quickly after stopping the antibiotics.[29]

I met with a woman who had been to see four of the top Lyme doctors in the country. She had been on antibiotics for more than fourteen years and hospitalized multiple times with bad side effects. After one series of treatments from an adverse reaction to one of the antibiotics, she almost died. And after all of her treatment, she actually feels worse. Fortunately, these types of reactions are not common, but they do happen. And there is no way to know in advance who may be seriously affected by them. If you are thinking about taking long-term antibiotics to treat Lyme disease, be aware—the risk is real.

The International Lyme and Associated Diseases Society (ILADS) developed guidelines for treating Lyme disease that are radically different from the CDC recommendations.[30] Many ILADS physicians and healthcare providers recognize that current CDC guidelines do not reflect the true complexity of Lyme disease or address variations in individual responses to the infection. If you are working with an ILADS provider, discuss with them the risks and benefits of antibiotic therapy for you.

Your Immune System

Autoimmune diseases have steadily been on the rise worldwide over the past several decades.[31] Diseases such as lupus, rheumatoid arthritis, type 1 diabetes, Crohn's disease, multiple sclerosis, celiac disease, and Hashimoto's disease (hypothyroid) are known to be caused by an autoimmune process. (For a complete list, see Appendix C, page 334.) In fact, more than 120 different diseases are either known or suspected to be related to autoimmunity.[32] The increase in autoimmune disease almost parallels the rise in asthma and allergies, which are mostly seen in industrialized countries and rarely in third-world countries.[33]

This has led some scientists to theorize that all of the microbes with which humans easily coexisted in the past had a protective effect on the human immune system. Trying to eradicate infectious disease by sterilizing away all germs accidentally upset the balance in the body's microbes, causing them to lose their protective benefit. The immune systems now react to what used to be benign.

Since I took my first immunology class in 1987, we have learned a tremendous amount about how the immune system works. The immune system is a complicated network of cells, organs, and chemicals that "talk" to each other in ways we don't fully understand. Every part of the immune system plays an essential role in keeping foreign microbes and allergens from harming the body.

Highly organized, your immune system has been trained since before you were born to identify what is part of you and what is not. It knows what is "self" and what is "not self." Doctors call this *immune tolerance*, an important mechanism by which the immune system turns itself *on* during an infection and *off* when the infection clears. But when some people get exposed to certain toxins or infections, the immune system can begin to lose tolerance to "self." So everything that is part of the person—gut, joints, muscles, skin, and brain, for example—becomes an immune target for the first time. This is autoimmune disease. While many factors may cause autoimmune disease, infections, like Lyme, are often overlooked. Yet a growing body of evidence suggests that bacteria and viruses may sometimes cause the immune system to start working against itself.[34]

Each autoimmune disease affects each person differently, but the common thread is inflammation—inflammation that slowly destroys both bodily tissues and function. Although more than a hundred conditions are associated with autoimmune disease, this section describes some of the more common ones. Many have no known triggers—doctors don't know precisely what causes them. But the presence of one of these diseases suggests that Lyme disease or another infectious disease may be at the root of the problem.

Medicine can tell you exactly what is happening to your body—we can measure your level of inflammation, but without any real understanding of *why* it occurs. Why would the immune system randomly turn against its host without some trigger? If you consult with most rheumatologists (specialists in autoimmune diseases) and ask them why you have an autoimmune disease, they often shrug and say, "Frankly, I don't know." The lack of curiosity as to causes of health conditions has always bothered me.

The reality is, there are likely many causes of autoimmune problems, including the following:

- Diet
- Exposure to toxic chemicals
- Stress
- Leaky gut
- Overuse or long-term use of certain medications
- Infection with certain microbes

As a former microbiologist, I have always been fascinated with how various bugs cause disease in the body. Upon exposure, some people get no symptoms at all, while others with the same exposure become deathly ill. Why? What is the difference between those who do and do not get sick when they are equally exposed? In my experience, the answer lies within the immune system.

Infection, Autoimmunity, and Molecular Mimicry

The cause of autoimmunity is mostly due to *molecular mimicry*. This occurs when an invading microbe has proteins that are similar to those found on your own cells. The result? Your immune system, unable to tell the difference between what is foreign and what is part of you, gets confused and attacks both. This results in antibodies accidentally attaching to parts of your body, creating inflammation and destruction in your organs and tissues.

To make matters worse, most doctors won't regard infection as a cause of your symptoms if you don't have the symptoms typically associated with that microbe. For example, if you have fatigue, high fever, swollen glands, and abdominal pain, your doctor will most likely look to see if you have been infected with Epstein-Barr virus, which causes mononucleosis (mono). However, if you have multiple sclerosis or lupus, your doctor would probably not test you for Epstein-Barr because you don't have the symptoms of mono. It's no secret that if you don't look for the cause, you'll never find it. Part of any doctor's obligation is to try to find out what makes you sick. If you have an autoimmune disease, make sure your doctor checks to see if an underlying infection is the root of your problem. Exposure to many of these infections can be determined through a simple blood test.

. . . .

Macrophages, T Cells, and Receptor Sites

The mechanisms by which microbes can cause autoimmunity are complicated and only partially understood. During a normal infection, large white blood cells called macrophages help your T cells make receptors on their cell surface that are specific to the microbe they are trying to fight. Think of receptors like a lock and key, where only one type of key will unlock a door. Each receptor is like a key that fits the lock on the surface of the microbe. This helps our immune system be very specific during an infection, so that T cells bind only to the foreign bug. In autoimmunity, though, scientists suggest that T cells accidentally make two receptors—one against the microbe and one against our own cells.[35] So as the immune system ramps up to kill the microbe, it attacks us in the process.

. . . .

Lyme Disease and Autoimmunity

Many symptoms seen with chronic or persistent Lyme can be attributed to autoimmunity. Genetics may also play a role in developing autoimmunity after getting Lyme disease. Research suggests that a protein found on the outer surface of the *Borrelia* bacterium, called outer-surface protein A (OspA), is structurally similar to a protein in our body (human lymphocyte function associated antigen-1 or hLFA-1).[36] This is what causes people with Lyme disease to develop joint pain, even if they have been treated with antibiotics. While these names don't mean anything to you, to immunologists and doctors, they signify that Lyme disease can trick the immune system into attacking the joints.

Multiple other proteins also cross-react with the Lyme organism, including endothelial cell growth factor (ECGF), apolipoprotein B-100, and annexin A2—which are commonly found in people with other autoimmune diseases, such as rheumatoid arthritis and lupus.[37] One study found that antibodies directed against the tail (called the *flagellum*) of the Lyme disease bacterium cross-react with a protein in the nerves that go to your arms and legs, causing numbness, tingling, and pain.[38] There is also evidence that Lyme-reactive antibodies form against proteins in the brain, giving rise to neurological symptoms.[39] With so many different proteins in your organs and cells that your immune system can confuse with Lyme disease, it's no wonder so many people with Lyme disease end up with long-term autoimmune problems.

Not all scientists agree that Lyme causes an autoimmune disease, but most research shows that it does. As a practicing physician, I regularly see that people with autoimmune disease and those with Lyme disease share strikingly similar signs and symptoms.

Although antibiotic therapy tries to kill only the bug, it does not support the immune system. So if Lyme has already triggered an autoimmune reaction in your body, continuing to try to kill the bug doesn't help you regain immune system health. Moreover, antibiotics devastate your gut flora.

To get your immune system back on track, you need to start with the most basic foundation of your health—your gut. That's why the Immune-Boosting Plan in Chapter 3 begins with gut health. Second, in all phases of the plan, you will reduce the load on the immune system so that it can recover. Here's a quick overview that shows the difference between my program and the all too common antibiotic treatments:

- Antibiotics kill the microbe but fail to address the autoimmunity that the microbe triggers. My program intervenes to alter the autoimmune response.
- Antibiotics can suppress your innate immune system, making it harder to fight the infection on your own. My program engages your natural immune-fighting ability to do what it is designed to do.
- Antibiotics accidentally kill off your normal flora in your gut, mouth, throat, skin, vagina . . . everywhere. These microbes are necessary for normal immune function and help protect you against other infections. By destroying your microbiome, you damage your own immune defenses.

- Antibiotics have many side effects. My program is well tolerated, with few to no side effects, so it can be used long-term in both adults and children.

In addition to other complications of antibiotic treatment, most Lyme antibiotics are so acidic they undermine full (and in many cases *any*) recovery from Lyme. Before you start up with what can turn out to be years of antibiotics, try these approaches first. People with Lyme disease need an orientation to the shape-shifting world of Lyme and concrete recommendations, based on the best and most inclusive treatment approach. That is what this book will provide.

One of the tenets of naturopathic medicine is *Vis Medicatrix Naturae*, "the healing power of nature." Naturopathic doctors like me recognize that the human body has a wisdom that inherently seeks to heal. It is in our DNA. But sometimes things block that process. This book can help you and your doctor find out what is stopping you from getting well and use the most effective, least harmful ways to facilitate your healing.

As much as you want to keep getting better each and every day, the road out of Lyme disease has its bumps and hiccups. You will have tough days. You will have good days. You will have days when you fight for the strength to push ahead. But you are a warrior and have resilience. You are tougher than you think, fighting the good fight. This is you, your health, and your life. Let's get started.

CHAPTER 2

How Do You Know If You Have Lyme?

This chapter looks at how you can find out if you have Lyme disease. What are the signs and symptoms? The Lyme Disease Symptom Questionnaire (page 42) will tell you how likely it is that you fit the profile of someone with Lyme disease. You will also learn about the available tests for Lyme disease. How good are they? Which ones should you take, and why?

As you will learn in this chapter, the various forms of tests available are, to put it mildly, anywhere from imperfect to useless. As a result, at just the time when you most need medical answers, you are unlikely to get them. This can be exasperating and upsetting when so much has already changed in your life due to this illness. I feel for you—I've been there. That is why I designed this chapter to both orient you to what's out there, so that you can make sense of any test results you've received so far, and to offer some basic guidance going forward from here and now.

Signs and Symptoms

In the complex world of Lyme, many people believe there is at least one certainty. If nothing else, you can rely on that well-known sign that you have been bitten by a Lyme tick—the telltale bull's-eye rash, the red ring that develops around the bite.

Or can you?

The bull's-eye rash is reliable proof that you have been bitten by a Lyme tick, but some individuals with Lyme develop a different kind of rash, or none at all. The CDC states that 70 to 80 percent of people with Lyme disease get the bull's-eye rash.[1] However, other experts in the field feel this number is grossly exaggerated and that the rash may only be seen in up to 50 percent of people who get Lyme disease.[2] Joint swelling, another sign of Lyme disease, is not a reliable gauge either, since it is found in only about 30 percent of people.[3] The fact is, people in early-stage Lyme experience a wide variety of symptoms.

Lyme may present itself as a flu-like illness. You may get fever, chills, sweats, and muscle aches. Or you may feel fatigue. Other than the bull's-eye rash, there is no single, unmistakable sign that you have Lyme bacteria in your system at this early stage.

JOHN'S STORY

When John came to my clinic, he told me that he had had chronic arthritis and significant back pain for more than twenty years. He also complained of chronic fatigue, muscle pain, and headaches. John had been to more than a dozen doctors and specialists and had been diagnosed with chronic fatigue syndrome and fibromyalgia. To help relieve his symptoms, his doctors prescribed multiple painkillers and muscle relaxants. But while these drugs helped somewhat to control his pain, their many side effects interfered with his daily life and work. When I began working with John, his blood tests for autoimmune diseases like rheumatoid arthritis and lupus were all negative. The only tests that repeatedly came back positive were the ones for inflammatory markers—these were always elevated.

I asked John if he had ever been tested for Lyme disease. He told me that he had been living in Florida, where his doctors did not believe Lyme disease existed and so refused to test him for Lyme. But his doctors neglected to ask him where he grew up, which happened to be Connecticut—a state with one of the highest rates of infection from Lyme disease!

I recommended he get a Lyme screen test through his local reference laboratory, A widely available test, and the one most doctors offer first, this test looks for specific Lyme antibodies. In John's case, the results were negative. However, as I well knew from my work as a microbiologist in a clinical laboratory (before I became a physician), this test often produces false negatives. A false negative means that the person *has* the disorder but the test reports that they don't. Knowing that is a common result with this particular test, I decided to run a more sensitive and specific antibody test called a Lyme Western blot. The guideline from the CDC is to first run the screening test. I often don't run the screening test because it is so faulty, but since it's the CDC protocol, many doctors offer this test. Later, I will discuss this issue in greater depth.

When I ran the more accurate Western blot, John's results came back positive. My suspicions had been confirmed: John was very likely exposed to a tick bite and infected with Lyme disease when he was living in Connecticut and had never been properly diagnosed. Once I knew what was causing his symptoms, he started the same treatment you will follow in this book. Within six weeks, almost all of his symptoms had resolved. It has now been almost two years since his diagnosis. I am happy to report that John is living symptom-free.

The Great Imitator

John's case clearly shows why Lyme disease has become so problematic: many who are infected are never diagnosed. Many others are diagnosed incorrectly. In fact, I refer to Lyme disease as "the Great Imitator," since it can look like many other illnesses. This often tempts health-care providers to look for other diseases, when the problem *is* actually Lyme. I am always saddened to hear about a person who has complained for years of Lyme-like symptoms but has gone untested because their doctor felt it was unnecessary. This oversight is bad enough if the patient lives in an area where Lyme disease is uncommon. But when it happens where Lyme disease is epidemic, it's alarming.

To make matters worse, doctors receive little education on Lyme disease in medical school. It is only when physicians get into clinical practice and start seeing Lyme in all of its various manifestations that they begin to understand it. This is why, when you consult a doctor, you must be your own best advocate. If your doctor or health-care provider resists testing you, then find someone who will. Every practitioner who treats Lyme disease knows that the sooner you start treatment, the better your chances of recovery. (See the Resources section, page 325, for a guide to practitioners.)

Meet the Spirochetes

In the United States, there are more than a hundred species of *Borrelia*. Worldwide, there are more than three hundred species, though not all species make people sick. Even though most people associate Lyme disease with a tick, it's actually a little more complicated than that. What causes Lyme disease in one part of the country (or world) may be different from what causes infection somewhere else. We know that *Borrelia burgdorferi* is the most common cause of Lyme disease on the East Coast of the United States, but *Borrelia miyamotoi* accounts for up to half of all infections on the West Coast. The types of *Borrelia* that cause Lyme disease found in Europe and Asia are different strains altogether. Some of the more well-known bacteria that cause Lyme disease include the following:

- *Borrelia burgdorferi*: This was the first strain identified as causing Lyme disease. It accounts for most cases in the United States.
- *Borrelia miyamotoi*: This is the second most common strain of *Borrelia* in the United States. It's most typically found on the West Coast but is also sometimes seen in East Coast ticks.[4]
- *Borrelia garinii*: The most common European strain of Lyme disease, it seems to cause more neurological symptoms than other strains of Lyme disease.[5]
- *Borrelia afzelii*: This strain is also found primarily in Europe; the symptoms that typically arise from it are usually localized in the skin.[6]

- *Borrelia mayonii*: One of the newest U.S. species to cause Lyme disease, this strain seems to be limited to seven states within the Midwest.[7]
- *Borrelia lonestari*: This yet-to-be-identified organism is the presumptive cause of southern tick-associated rash illness (STARI), a disease almost identical to Lyme disease found in the southeastern and south-central United States. Several differences between STARI and Lyme disease are that the rash associated with this strain isn't as big, the symptoms are milder, and the condition usually responds well to antibiotics.[8]

Lyme disease can be divided into two stages, acute and chronic. The symptoms at each stage can look very different, though there is some overlap.

As you know, the first and most important symptom is the bull's-eye rash. Technically called *erythema chronicum migrans* (literally, "chronic red spreading"), this is the telltale sign of acute Lyme. It usually occurs in the early stage of infection at the site of the tick bite. I have heard from countless people who were told by doctors that they didn't have Lyme disease because they never developed it.[9] I am repeating this crucial point because it's likely you have been told that very same thing. But it isn't true. Remember, even without a bull's-eye rash you still may have been exposed.

But if you do develop the classic rash, you can be certain that a tick bite *has* transmitted Lyme disease. The bull's-eye rash is Lyme specific. All the other symptoms of acute Lyme disease listed earlier may or may not occur, but they are not specific to Lyme disease and can reflect any number of other types of illnesses.

If You've Been Bitten by a Deer Tick

If you have been bitten by a deer tick, or suspect you have, especially if you live in an area where ticks are common, what should you do? First, of course, remove the tick and clean the bite area with soap and water or isopropyl alcohol. Instructions on how to remove a tick are on page 45. Then, immediately start the Immune-Boosting Diet on page 88 of this book. Follow the diet until a tick test or your own blood test comes back negative.

If you notice the bite within the first seventy-two hours, and you are an adult, please get antibiotic treatment immediately. This is the one instance in which I positively recommend a dose of antibiotics. Lyme disease responds to early detection and treatment. In addition, carefully monitor your symptoms after a bite, as they can take up to thirty days to develop. I recommend taking children who may have received a tick bite to see a pediatrician or health-care provider who can discuss the options for getting early treatment.

The bottom line is that diagnosing early-stage Lyme disease can be tricky.

- You may get a tick bite and not know you have been bitten.
- You may get bitten and know it, but not realize you have been infected.
- You may or may not develop a bull's-eye rash.
- If your early-stage symptoms are mild, you or your physician may attribute them to some other bacterial or viral infection and go without any kind of treatment for Lyme at all.

Chronic Lyme Disease

If left untreated, as time goes on, the Lyme infection can become progressively worse, with a variety of symptoms. Among the more than forty symptoms associated with chronic Lyme disease, some of the most common are the following:

- Wandering joint pain (moves frequently from joint to joint)
- Brain fog and forgetfulness
- Insomnia
- Chronic swollen glands
- Unexplained fever or sweating
- Chronic fatigue
- Mood swings and irritability
- Depression
- Muscle twitching
- Ringing in ears (tinnitus)
- Heart palpitations
- Irritable bowel syndrome
- Thyroid problems (usually hypothyroid)
- Changes in handwriting and mixing up words
- Sexual function problems

This is a formidable list, and a good reason to deal with Lyme disease early and effectively.

Clinical Diagnosis

Because there is no simple, definitive test for Lyme disease, physicians use what is known as a *clinical diagnosis*. That means it is based on both your exposure to deer ticks and your signs and symptoms—and not on a laboratory test alone. Current methods of testing can help confirm a diagnosis, but to be perfectly frank, they are not reliable enough by themselves to tell whether you have Lyme disease. To arrive at a diagnosis, it is best to look at symptoms combined with tests. Let's see why it's essential to approach your diagnosis in this way.

ERIN'S STORY

Erin was a delightful eight-year-old, born and raised in upstate New York. Her mother brought her to our clinic because she had started developing facial tics. Other than the tics, she was a healthy child. All the tests run by her pediatrician came back normal. But the tics were worsening and becoming more frequent. When I asked if Erin had ever been tested for Lyme disease, her mother told me that her pediatrician would not order the test since she did not have symptoms of Lyme disease.

Since streptococcus bacteria are a common cause of tics, I ordered tests for strep and Lyme. The strep test came back negative, but her Lyme test came back positive. Erin did not display many of the other symptoms common in people with Lyme disease, but it was clearly a cause of her tics. At her mom's request, we started her on herbal therapy and immunotherapy. Her tics started to go away almost immediately. After two months of treatment, they disappeared, and she was back to being a healthy, happy child.

Erin's case reveals that people with Lyme disease may fail to develop every one of its numerous symptoms. This complex illness can manifest in many different ways. Some people experience only a few symptoms. Others can be completely debilitated. If your doctor is looking only for classic Lyme disease, he or she is going to miss most people who actually have it. This is a frustrating and puzzling experience for many people with Lyme disease. Fortunately, I have some ways to help.

THE LYME DISEASE SYMPTOM QUESTIONNAIRE

If you do not develop a bull's-eye rash, getting a Lyme disease diagnosis can be complicated. I'll explain more about this later in the chapter. Meanwhile, there are a few things you can and should do while you wait to get tested or seek out a Lyme-literate doctor.

I've developed a quick and easy questionnaire to help you assess the likelihood that you have Lyme disease. I am offering it right here, early in the chapter, even before taking up the question of testing. Why? Because with or without a visible bite, it's urgent that you learn to identify Lyme's characteristic symptoms right away. Once you have your results, if you do have Lyme disease, you can begin treatment as soon as possible—before the disease progresses. You can also retake the questionnaire periodically during treatment as a gauge of your results on *The Lyme Solution* plan. I encourage you to share your answers with your doctor. Knowledge of your current symptoms will help him or her manage your care.

Although the questionnaire is only a first step, it's an important one in finding out how likely it is that you have Lyme disease. The questions align with the approach of the International Lyme and Associated Diseases Society (ILADS), a group of physicians who advocate for less reliance on testing. They prefer to use a person's own signs and symptoms along with the history of possible exposure to determine the likelihood that someone has Lyme disease. (At any time, of course, you can also consult your health-care provider.) To take the questionnaire, for each symptom, insert a number from 0 to 4 in the severity column. A scoring key follows the test. If you have the characteristic bull's-eye rash, then it is almost certain you have Lyme disease and you can skip the questionnaire.

SYMPTOM SCORE
- 0 = None
- 1 = Rare
- 2 = Mild
- 3 = Moderate
- 4 = Severe

SYMPTOM	SEVERITY
Fever, chills, or sweating	
Joint pain or swelling in multiple joints	
Numbness, tingling, or burning pain	
Muscle pain or twitching	
Muscle weakness	
Bell's palsy or facial paralysis	
Hand tremors	
Chronic fatigue	
Chronic swollen glands	
Chronic constipation or diarrhea	
Forgetfulness or memory loss	
Headaches	
Dizziness or light-headedness	
Changes in vision (blurry or double vision)	
Insomnia	
Ringing in the ears	
Shortness of breath	
Heart palpitations	
Irritable bladder	
Loss of libido	

SYMPTOM	SEVERITY
Sudden change in mood	
Sudden change in handwriting or speech	
Add 4 points if you live or have been in an area where Lyme disease is common.	
Add 4 points if you have been diagnosed with another autoimmune illness.	
TOTAL	

HOW TO SCORE THE QUESTIONNAIRE

If your score is less than 20, it is unlikely that you have Lyme disease. If your score is between 21 and 44, it is possible that you have been exposed to an infected tick, and you should:

- Start the Immune-Boosting Diet in Chapter 4, if you have not started already.
- Get tested by a physician who is familiar with the approach to Lyme disease offered in this book (see the Resources section, page 325, for a list of recommended practitioners).

If your score is over 45, or if you have a bull's-eye rash, it is highly likely you have Lyme disease or some other tick-borne illness, and you should:

- Start the Immune-Boosting Diet in Chapter 4.
- Begin the advanced protocols in Chapter 3.
- Get tested by a physician who is familiar with the approach to Lyme disease offered in this book (see the Resources section for a list of recommended practitioners).

What to Do If You Find a Tick

There are many types of ticks in various regions of this country. Not all of them carry Lyme disease. And those that do are so small that unless a Lyme-carrying tick is already engorged with blood, it can be very difficult to see without a magnifying glass. If you happen to have a lot of hair on your skin, spotting ticks is even more difficult. The first time I actually found a tick on my body, I thought it was just a small fleck of dirt on my arm until I saw it move as I tried to scratch it off.

Get in the habit of doing a tick check on yourself and your family if you have spent any time outdoors—especially if you have been in the woods, playing on grass, gardening, or doing other activities where you are around a lot of trees or plants. If you live in a Lyme-endemic area, get to know the various tick types, so you can identify the difference between a deer tick and other varieties.

How to Remove a Tick

If you find a tick on your own or your child's body:

1. Get a pair of fine-tipped tweezers and grab the tick as close to your skin as possible. I like tweezers that have a small magnifying glass attached to them, so you can see what you're doing better. Slowly lift straight up on the tick until you feel it come out of your skin. Use slow, gentle pressure. Do not twist or pull, as you may break off parts of the tick by accident. If you take your time, you can usually remove the whole tick without breaking it. If the tick does break, try to grab the pieces left in your skin with your

tweezers. If you can't grab them, then just wash the area thoroughly with soap and water and your skin will naturally expel the leftover pieces in a few days.

2. Once the tick is removed, place it in a Ziploc bag with a moist cotton ball. The moisture will help preserve the tick until it can be tested. If you wish to discard the tick, put it in a sealed bag and dispose of it, flush it down the toilet, or put it in a small glass of rubbing alcohol for twenty-four hours. The latter method will kill the tick and then it can be safely discarded. Do not use your fingers to try to crush it.

3. Wash the area of the bite well with a disinfectant soap, hydrogen peroxide, iodine, or rubbing alcohol.

4. Take a picture of the area where the bite occurred, so you can document how the skin changes. If you develop a bull's-eye rash, it may continue to get larger over the course of many weeks.

What Next?

To be safe, once you've removed the tick or if you think you've been bitten by one:

1. Go on the Immune-Boosting Diet in Chapter 4.

2. See your health-care provider and start antibiotic therapy within seventy-two hours of the tick bite.

3. Take Coptis, an herb that can sometimes help eradicate the tickborne microbes before symptoms appear. Adults should take two capsules three times per day after initial infection and taper down to one capsule three times per day after three to four weeks. Children older than eight years old should take one capsule three

times per day. For children younger than eight years old, please consult your health-care provider to discuss treatment options. (For more information about Coptis, see page 139.)

4. Have the tick tested for Lyme disease and co-infections. Many labs do tick testing, some faster than others. (See the Resources section, page 325.) The lab I use, Medical Diagnostic Laboratories (Hamilton, New Jersey) gets results within a few days. A negative tick test does not guarantee that Lyme disease cannot develop, but it is rare in my experience for someone to develop Lyme if the tick was negative on testing. You can use other labs or your state public health department, but they are very slow in getting results.

5. Monitor your symptoms closely for the month following a tick bite. If there is any indication that you are starting to develop any of the symptoms of Lyme disease, then follow the guidelines in this book for:

> Targeting active infection through natural herbs and other substances (Chapter 5)
> Transforming your immediate surroundings to support immune system health (Chapter 6)
> Following the advanced protocols (Chapter 8)
> Cycling back through the program as needed (Chapter 9)

Lyme Disease Testing: No Reliable Tests

Although this book recommends various blood tests for Lyme, it's important to bear in mind that unfortunately there are no tests that can give a definitive diagnosis. A bacterial culture—which entails growing bacteria in a petri dish in a laboratory—is the gold standard for diagnosing bacterial infections. This is the best way to positively identify an organism. But to date, the Lyme organism has been difficult to culture. There is no accepted method of doing this. Researchers also don't know what specimen (blood, urine, tissue) is best for capturing Lyme disease, since it can invade so many different areas of the body. The best we have are antibody tests, which merely reflect your immune system reacting to the infection. Since the normal immune response is to make antibodies against a bacterial infection, the presence of antibodies alone reveals only that you have been exposed to Lyme disease. It does not tell us whether you have Lyme disease. It shows only that your immune system did what it is supposed to do—try to fight off the infection. The only truly accurate method for determining the presence of Lyme disease is tissue biopsy and culture, but this technique is so invasive, it is never done in routine clinical practice. Other current tests can miss up to 60 percent of Lyme cases.[10]

In fact, some physicians regard current tests for Lyme completely worthless, since some of the tested antibodies are not Lyme specific, and some that they do *not* test for are. One reason for this problem is that the CDC does not recognize all of the Lyme-specific antibodies (largely for political reasons, but that's a discussion for another time). Fortunately, many good labs do. Lyme researchers Dr. Raphael Stricker and Lorraine Johnson have referred to currently available tests for the Lyme spirochete as no more effective than tossing a coin![11]

So why use them at all? Well, if a test comes back positive, then at least you know that you have been exposed to Lyme disease, as there are very few false-positive results. However, if your test comes back negative, you cannot rule out the possibility that you have Lyme disease.

Two-Stage Testing

The CDC's current recommendation for someone suspected of having Lyme disease is a two-stage test. The first stage is a Lyme antibody blood test known as the ELISA (enzyme-linked immunosorbent assay), or the Lyme screen test. The second test is a different antibody test called the Lyme Western blot test, or the Western blot for short.

The Lyme Screen Test

The Lyme screen test measures two types of antibodies against Lyme disease, immunoglobulin G (IgG) and immunoglobulin M (IgM). In response to an infection, the immune system produces *immunoglobulins*, which are antibodies. By attaching themselves to the bacteria or virus, these antibodies alert the immune system that something foreign has penetrated the body. Once the antibodies attach to the bug, other parts of the immune system can then eradicate the infection.

IgM is usually the first antibody your immune system sends in after you are exposed to a microbe. As a result, for more typical kinds of infections, if you take an IgM test and get positive results, they signify that you have a recent exposure to the infection. In contrast, an IgG response kicks in at later stages of the illness or infection. So if you take the IgG test and get a positive result, that suggests you have an older or past infection. But in looking to diagnose Lyme disease via antibody-based tests like the Lyme screen test, all bets are off.

One study found that in fifty-five people with known Lyme disease, less than 46 percent of them had either IgG or IgM antibodies when first tested.[12] And I have seen people in exactly the opposite situation—with IgM antibodies from years prior and IgG antibodies from a recent exposure. The bottom line is that if you take the Lyme screen test today, there is absolutely no guarantee that it will distinguish between active and past infection. In other words, don't rely on it to determine when you were exposed to an infected tick.

Even in terms of what it's *supposed* to do, the Lyme screen test isn't very sensitive. A good screening test should pick up at least 95 percent of the people who have the condition the test is used for, according to the College of American Pathologists. The Lyme screen test does not meet these criteria.[13] In fact, the Lyme screen test may pick up only about 56 percent of people who have Lyme disease.[14] To make matters worse, since the CDC guidelines do not recommend doing a Western blot (the second test) if the Lyme screen is negative, a doctor may easily skip doing the Western blot, which is a more sensitive and specific test. Research shows that the Western blot is more accurate in diagnosing Lyme disease because it looks for specific antibodies often seen in people with Lyme disease but not found in healthy controls.[15] I rarely run the Lyme screen on people I suspect have Lyme disease and go straight to the Western blot to get better information.

The Western Blot

The second stage of the CDC's recommended two-stage test is the Western blot. This test doesn't detect the Lyme bacteria itself. Instead, it detects any antibodies that may be present to fight off the Lyme spirochete. But since antibodies can hang around for years, even decades, the presence of antibodies does not necessarily mean there is a current infection.

The Western blot is also highly prone to false negatives. In other words, the test results reveal no antibodies even though there *is* a current infection. This occurs because it can take weeks for your body to develop antibodies against Lyme. That is why the CDC does not recommend doing a Western blot test on anyone whose illness occurred within the previous month.

CHRIS'S STORY

Chris came into my office five years ago complaining of joint pain and numbness in his hands and feet that had been ongoing for about a week. He also had a mild headache that just didn't seem to go away. When I examined him, I noticed a bull's-eye rash on his shoulder. He told me he thought it was just a mosquito bite. Chris is an avid outdoorsman and spends a lot of his free time hunting and fishing, so he said he gets bitten often by mosquitoes in the summer and has pulled several ticks off his skin over the years.

Given his bull's-eye rash, he likely had received a tick bite and had Lyme disease. And sure enough, when I did the Lyme screen through our local laboratory, his test came back positive. But when I ran the follow-up Lyme Western blot, it came back negative. I went ahead and started Chris on treatment based on his clinical symptoms and the bull's-eye rash, and after several weeks he started to improve. I ran the tests again after four weeks. This time both the Lyme screen and the Western blot were positive. Chris's earlier Western blot result was probably negative because his exposure had been fairly recent. His body had not yet launched a full immune response. His case reveals why the timing of the tests is important.

More Issues with the Western Blot

There's another problem with the Western blot. Many people who end up with chronic Lyme disease do not have a healthy immune system to start with. Therefore they do not produce enough antibodies either to get rid of the infection or to show up on a test. So even if the body's immune system does respond, the response may be too weak for the test to notice. To add yet another wrinkle, antibody levels can also fluctuate over time, for reasons that are not well understood. I have seen this in hundreds of people who have taken the Western blot test.

No wonder the Western blot misses up to 60 percent of cases of early-stage Lyme disease! With this test, retesting is often required.

Yet another difficulty is that the criteria used to call a Western blot test "positive" are thirty years old![16] The Western blot looks primarily for one strain of the common Lyme spirochete, *Borrelia burgdorferi*, although many cases of Lyme disease, on the West Coast of the United States in particular and in other parts of the world, are caused by entirely different types of *Borrelia*, which do *not* get picked up on the test. The standard Lyme screen and Western blot test run by most reference labs only look for *Borrelia burgdorferi* and do not test for other types of *Borrelia*.

Fortunately, other specialty labs such as Medical Diagnostic Laboratories (Hamilton, New Jersey) and IGeneX (Palo Alto, California) do offer more comprehensive testing for other strains of *Borrelia* known to cause Lyme disease. They include *Borrelia miyamotoi*, *Borrelia afzelii*, *Borrelia garinii*, and *Borrelia lonestari*. Not all antibodies tested by the Western blot are specific for Lyme disease. In fact, some of the antibodies will react to other microbes unrelated to Lyme. For example, the 31kD antibody on the Western blot can show up positive in someone who has Epstein-Barr virus, the cause of mono. So if someone had mono, it would cause that specific antibody to be positive on the test but does not mean that the person has Lyme disease. Once again, you can see that the test recommended by the CDC is woefully outdated and inadequate.

Finally, while there are agreed-to ways to determine a positive or negative result, the Western blot lacks official guidelines for borderline test results. In many Western blot test results, the people tested have only four out of ten IgG antibodies instead of the five out of ten required to call the test positive. The CDC states that two of three IgM antibodies need to be present to call the test positive, but although you may have only one out of three antibodies for IgM, that one antibody is Lyme specific. In other words, the tests assume that each person exposed to *Borrelia* has the same exact immune response—but that is never the case. The CDC's strict criteria fail to recognize the diversity of immune responses among human beings. If someone does have several Lyme-specific antibodies, even if they do not meet the CDC criteria, isn't that important? It's kind of like being a *little* pregnant.

By this point, you may be wondering whether you should even bother to take the test. If so, when to take it? How should you (or your doctor) interpret the results you receive, given all the inconsistencies in test results?

I recommend the following if your symptom picture or a bull's-eye rash suggests that you have Lyme disease:

Do the Lyme Western blot—preferably with a lab (like those I mentioned earlier) that specializes in comprehensive Lyme testing. I advise that you also test for co-infections, so you know exactly what you're dealing with as you go forward in your treatment. If your doctor is resistant to getting you tested properly, find a doctor who will (see the Resources section, page 325, to find a Lyme-literate doctor).

I have seen enough of these tests to realize that people with Lyme disease symptoms who have borderline tests, especially when they have Lyme-specific antibodies, respond well to the Immune-Boosting Plan. Although the Lyme Western blot is not a perfect test, I still run it with anyone suspected of having Lyme disease, as a positive test would confirm my diagnosis. But if the test comes back negative, it does not exclude the possibility of Lyme disease. Despite the reliability issues with all Lyme testing, it is still worth doing, as it is the best test we currently have to help identify whether you've been exposed to Lyme.

LORI'S STORY

An Australian woman came to my clinic when she was in the United States on a business trip. Her medical history included chronic fatigue, sleep problems, brain fog, poor strength and stamina, joint pain, head pressure, dizziness, and stomach problems, to name just some of her many symptoms. Working with several practitioners in Sydney, she had undergone various natural treatments with only slight progress. In our consultation, I reviewed her whole health history.

Her previous lab work revealed elevated inflammatory markers, such as an erythrocyte sedimentation rate (ESR) and C-reactive protein (CRP), which I discuss on page 240. But neither lab results nor doctors could interpret this important clue about Lori's actual health issue. When I asked if her local doctor had tested her for Lyme disease, the answer was no.

Timely Lyme treatment requires a Lyme-savvy local health-care system. The Australian government's policy is that Lyme disease does not exist there. In seeking out the right diagnosis and treatment, Lori faced a health-care system in denial. In keeping with this unscientific policy decision, the Australian medical system routinely fails to find *Borrelia* (the most prevalent Lyme spirochete) in any of the ticks they have tested. But they have only been testing ticks for *Borrelia burgdorferi*, which we know is the common type in North America but not necessarily in Australia. It is likely that they are just looking for the wrong bug.

Even if no one in Australia could possibly contract Lyme disease, an absurd notion since Lyme-infected deer ticks are found everywhere, many citizens like Lori and her husband are avid travelers. They, like many Australians, have been in parts of the world that are known to have Lyme disease. Her local doctors refused to account for her frequent trips out of the country to places where she could have picked up an infection.

Given the often iffy results of Lyme disease testing, her test results did not confirm a diagnosis. When Lori took the Western blot test using a U.S. lab, the result was only borderline positive. Nevertheless, we both suspected that she had been infected years ago during her travels. And her symptoms were also consistent with Lyme. Adding further weight to this conclusion, other illnesses had already been excluded.

Lori started an aggressive treatment of herbs, nutritional support, immune support, and detoxification therapies. We set up a plan she could also follow when she returned to Australia, and I found a local provider there to continue her care.

She has been following the treatment plan for more than a year now and her health is much improved. Her energy and brain fog are much better. She is able to do more physical activity. She has less joint pain, and her gut has been much happier. Fortunately, she has made great strides toward regaining her health.

What happened to Lori is all too common among people who miss getting an early diagnosis and receiving prompt treatment. When they try to play catch-up later, their odds of getting an accurate diagnosis, not to mention an effective treatment, aren't good. This is a high-risk factor for everyone in our Lyme-ignorant health-care system. But it's even worse for those who live where Lyme disease supposedly does not exist. The lack of medical know-how and testing cost Lori many precious years of good health. Do not let what happened to Lori happen to you. If you suspect Lyme disease, address it right away. Go on the Immune-Boosting Plan in this book. Get tested. And find a healthcare provider who will help you find the right answers.

Other Lyme-Helpful Tests

The CDC recommends only the two-step testing using the Lyme screen and the Western blot. As you have seen, these tests are unreliable when used on their own. That is why I want to recommend that you consider several other tests that can help determine exposure to Lyme bacteria.

POLYMERASE CHAIN REACTION (PCR)

Polymerase chain reaction (PCR) testing looks for small fragments of Lyme DNA in either the blood, urine, joint fluid, or cerebrospinal fluid. This can be helpful when the antibody response has been too small to pick up on standard Lyme screen or Western blot tests or when there may be only a small number of Lyme organisms in the body. The advantage of PCR testing for Lyme disease is that it is highly specific to the *Borrelia* species.

PCR testing is also useful because it lets you test any body fluid. This can be particularly helpful for someone who may have Lyme disease in the brain, since it can show whether the fluid around the brain is infected. Doctors can also use this test to find out if Lyme disease is causing a person's arthritis or swollen joints.

The disadvantage of PCR testing is that it is not very sensitive. Studies show that less than 50 percent of people with active Lyme disease have a positive PCR test.[17] This number goes down if they have been treated with antibiotics. Since there may be a low number of Lyme bacteria in the blood to begin with, antibiotics further decrease how much bacteria is detectable. Increased levels of IgG may actually interfere with the PCR test.[18] The other disadvantage is that it does not reveal whether the detected *Borrelia* are alive or dead. In short, a positive test does not necessarily indicate an active infection, and a negative test does not necessarily rule out prior or current exposure to *Borrelia*.

Given these parameters, you may well wonder why I mention this test. I used to run this test often, until I saw that most of the tests were coming back negative, so I rarely order it anymore. While PCR testing may be valuable in certain cases, such as using PCR on spinal fluid to determine whether someone has Lyme in the brain, I don't think it is helpful in trying to determine whether you have active Lyme disease. If it is recommended for you, remember that the PCR test is of limited use only.

BLOOD CULTURE

Culturing bacteria has been the gold standard for microbiology testing for decades. Once scientists can get bacteria to grow in a petri dish, identifying those bacteria is easy. Bacteria culturing has allowed microbiologists to be much more specific in their reports of what is causing infection.

Once again, however, Lyme disease is a special case, because it is difficult to grow the spirochetes outside the body. One reason is that *Borrelia* grows very, very slowly. Blood cultures pick up only 40 percent of cases of acute Lyme disease. That percentage is even lower for those with chronic Lyme.[19] When body fluids like joint or cerebrospinal fluid are tested, even among these with Lyme, positive tests are rare.

Until there are improvements in our ability to culture Lyme disease, this won't be an especially useful test for Lyme.

T CELL ACTIVATION TESTING

One of the newest tests—the Elispot from Armin Labs—measures T cell activation. T cells respond four to six days after an infection, while antibodies can take four weeks or longer to mobilize. This improves the odds of identifying Lyme in its early stages. For people who don't make antibodies against Lyme disease, this option can help determine whether Lyme disease is the culprit. This test looks at specific Lyme antigens, so false positives are unlikely.

Running both the Western blot and the T cell activation test can help you identify Lyme disease shortly after infection. This test can also help monitor treatment. The T cell test measures early-stage reactivity to Lyme disease. These levels will drop after you have been properly treated. Over the course of treatment, T cell activation test results often change from positive to negative.

The T cell test is helpful when someone's Lyme diagnosis is unclear. It can also be used during that early window before antibodies have formed. Talk with your health-care provider about whether this test may be right for you.

SUMMARY OF LYME TESTS

NAME		PURPOSE	UPSIDES AND DOWNSIDES
Two-Stage Test	*Lyme screen test*	Tests for IgG and IgM	Can't distinguish between active and past infection. Many false negatives. Limited to *Borrelia burgdorferi* only.
	Western blot test	Tests for Lyme antibodies	False negatives, especially if done too early; detects only free antibodies. Also limited to *Borrelia burgdorferi* only. A true positive test indicates exposure.
PCR		Tests for Lyme DNA	Useful for detecting Lyme in brain and other body fluids, but high false-negative rate. However, it is very specific, so a positive test indicates current exposure.
Blood culture		Tests for presence of Lyme bacteria	Low sensitivity, but a positive test indicates active infection with Lyme disease.
T cell activation test		Tests for specific T cell activity against Lyme	Not dependent on antibody responses, so useful in early Lyme disease or when antibody tests are questionable. False positives unlikely.

When It's Not Lyme Disease

There is an old saying that "If you only have a hammer, everything looks like a nail." This can be very true in the world of Lyme disease. While some doctors couldn't diagnose Lyme if they tripped over it, others want to believe that every symptom they find is related to Lyme.

An elderly woman once came to my office complaining of vulvodynia (pain in the groin) that her previous doctor had told her was Lyme disease requiring aggressive treatment. But three different tests were all negative. She had no other symptoms that suggested she had Lyme disease.

When I examined her, I noted a very red, inflamed rash in her groin area. I referred her to her gynecologist, who diagnosed a bad yeast infection that cleared up after antifungal therapy.

While most doctors I know who treat Lyme disease are diligent about looking at the whole person, some practitioners get tunnel vision and forget to rule out other possibilities—especially when a person tests negative. If you are symptomatic and all of your other tests have been normal, there may be a better explanation than Lyme disease for why you don't feel well.

This is not so surprising, since Lyme disease can resemble so many other conditions. In fact, more than three hundred conditions can mimic Lyme disease, including the following:

- Multiple sclerosis
- Rheumatoid arthritis
- Lupus
- Polymyalgia rheumatica

- Fibromyalgia
- Chronic fatigue syndrome
- Parkinson's disease
- Amyotrophic lateral sclerosis (ALS or Lou Gehrig's disease)
- Alzheimer's disease
- Mononucleosis (Mono)
- Depression
- Meningitis
- Small-intestine bacterial overgrowth (SIBO)
- Tourette's syndrome
- Irritable bowel syndrome (IBS)
- Migraines
- Restless legs syndrome (RLS)
- Vertigo

If on the basis of the Lyme Disease Symptom Questionnaire (page 42), or as a result of other testing, Lyme disease is ruled out in your case, your health-care provider may have to do some detective work to find out what's making you feel unwell. Getting the right information is the first step to health and wellness.

Putting It All Together

Your head may be spinning with all of this detailed information about Lyme testing. If you feel confused, you're not alone. Doctors and scientists have the same problems with all of these tests. None of them proves 100 percent that a person has Lyme disease. That's why it's best to keep in mind this one simple rule: Lyme tests can't prove that you have Lyme disease. All the Lyme tests are really just a way to confirm that you have been exposed to the Lyme organism.

Though it may be disconcerting to learn all about the shortfalls of each test, as I've detailed them in this chapter, please understand my purpose: to prepare you for the all-too-common scenario in which, despite your symptoms, you receive a negative test—and are told you don't have Lyme disease.

This happens constantly. People want to trust their doctors. But when it comes to Lyme disease, the tests are poor, and few doctors are sufficiently aware of all their pitfalls. Unless a doctor is extremely familiar with all of the reasons that a specific test might give a negative result, then he or she will often misinterpret the results—and misdiagnose you.

I recall one man who had five Western blot tests and all came back negative. But the sixth test came back positive, using the already low CDC standards. Fortunately, his doctor did not believe the previous five tests and had already started the man on treatment for Lyme disease.

I'm sure some of you reading this book have had experiences similar to this. For those of you who suspect you may have Lyme disease, it is important to work with a doctor or other health-care provider who really listens to your health concerns and who will run the right tests to help you find answers.

Your health-care provider needs to be diligent in finding the root of your illness. Another tenet of naturopathic medicine is *Tolle Causam*—"find the cause." It takes time to sort through someone's complex medical history, so make sure you are working with a provider who will take the time to help figure things out. If you are working with someone who refuses to treat your Lyme disease because you received an unreliable result, then you need to move on and find someone who will. Sometimes you have to be your own best advocate. It's no mystery that the sooner you start treatment, the sooner you will feel better. Ultimately, it is your health that is at stake.

Find the cause.

Start treatment.

Feel better.

Part Two

The Five-Stage
Immune-Boosting
Plan

In Chapters 1 and 2, you saw just how widespread the Lyme disease epidemic is and learned about my unique approach to this disease. By treating chronic Lyme disease as an autoimmune disorder and avoiding the usual heavy doses of antibiotics, I have helped thousands of people free themselves from this debilitating illness. In this and the next five chapters, I will share this knowledge with you as I unfold my Immune-Boosting Plan.

This novel approach to Lyme really delivers. But be prepared—it's nothing like what most doctors tell people with Lyme disease. And again that's because the very protocol that conventional doctors routinely offer exacerbates Lyme symptoms and undermines your chance of long-term recovery from Lyme disease.

It's not just about killing the bacteria. Instead, you will learn how to mitigate the immune effects that the bacteria trigger. At every phase of the program, the goal is to reduce the load on the immune system so that it can recover. That is why the Immune-Boosting Plan that begins in Chapter 3 can be used both to treat Lyme disease and to reduce your risk of infection if you are bitten.

You will follow these stages of treatment:

1. Repairing your gut to strengthen your immune system
2. Following the Immune-Boosting Diet
3. Targeting active infection through natural herbs and other substances
4. Transforming your immediate surroundings to support immune system health
5. Reducing your stress level and getting more sleep and exercise

On the Immune-Boosting Plan, you will be removing stressors, eliminating microbes, and building up your body's healthy immune defense system.

CHAPTER 3

The Gut Protocol
That Restores Your
Immune System

Your Gut Is the Key to a
Healthier Immune System

Countless people with Lyme disease report years of poor gut health, with chronic diarrhea, constipation, gas, bloating, heartburn, reflux, and abdominal pain. I had a patient who had only one bowel movement a week, despite eating three to four times a day, and was told by his primary-care doctor that this was normal! I can assure you, it is not normal! These are all symptoms of a gut that isn't working at its best.

Many people with Lyme disease say that they had gastrointestinal problems even before they became sick, sometimes since they were very young. That's important information, because it suggests that their immune dysfunction began long before they ever contracted Lyme disease. If you had a poor-functioning gut prior to getting Lyme disease, it may have set the stage for you to be less able to fight the infection on your own, making you more prone to autoimmunity.

But not everybody with Lyme disease has gut issues before getting infected. I see plenty of people with normal, healthy gut function until *after* they either got Lyme disease or started treatment with antibiotics.

No matter when your gut problems started, you will want to fix them as quickly as possible to help improve your immune function. Lyme disease both causes and results from an undermined immune system.

Building on my Chapter 1 discussion of autoimmunity as core to Lyme disease treatment, this chapter offers an Immune-Boosting Gut Protocol that lays the foundation for decreasing immune system reactivity. Whether you have experienced gut symptoms for a long time or they began with your Lyme symptoms, following the Immune-Boosting Gut Protocol in this chapter and the Immune-Boosting Diet in Chapter 4 will give you relief. In Chapters 6 and 7, you will also learn how to manage your stress, lifestyle, and environment to improve your overall health—because along with a poor diet, these factors can lead to abnormal changes in intestinal microbes and inflammation.

Let's begin by repairing your gut (in this chapter) and using the nutritional interventions I offer (in Chapter 4). Together, these steps will create an environment hospitable to your microbiome—an environment that is in turn *in*hospitable to the Lyme bug.

Immunity Starts in the Gut

Naturopathic medicine regards a healthy gut as a cornerstone of well-being. The gut plays a key role in making sure the body is nourished by food. By digesting your food and absorbing its nutrients into your bloodstream, your gut does the prep work and acts as a first-stage nutrient delivery system. The gut is also the largest organ in your immune system. It constitutes up to 80 percent of your body's immune function, protecting you from viruses, bacteria, and a host of chemicals and foreign bodies. The mouth, at one end of the digestive tract, is the main point of entry into the body, so it's no wonder your entire digestive tract from top to bottom is heavily involved in your body's defense system. Anything that alters normal digestive function adversely affects your immunity.

Signs Your Gut Is Unhappy

If your stomach and intestines work well, you will have regular, daily bowel movements with well-formed stool that is not loose, watery, or hard as a rock. You should feel that you digest your food well, without food repeating in you. But if you do start having gut problems, you may experience the following:

- Gas
- Bloating
- Constipation
- Diarrhea
- Heartburn
- Reflux
- Blood in your stool
- Mucus in your stool
- Undigested food in your stool
- Belching
- Flatulence
- Abdominal pain

Note: Blood in your stool can be a sign of internal bleeding, so if you ever see it, visit your doctor right away to find the cause.

There are many reasons your belly may be giving you trouble, which my program addresses. Eating highly processed foods, taking antibiotics or other medications, stress, or genetic conditions like celiac disease (gluten intolerance) can all lead to poor digestive health.[1] Using nonsteroidal anti-inflammatory drugs (NSAIDs) can also undermine digestive tract integrity. These problems don't happen overnight but develop over the course of weeks to years.

Good and Bad Bacteria

The fact that there are ten times as many bacteria in the body as actual human cells (we are literally 90 percent microbe!) tells you how important these organisms are to survival. The trillions of microbes that live in your gut are there for three reasons:[2]

1. To help keep "bad" bugs out and prevent infection.
2. To help maintain the intestinal barrier and increase secretory immunoglobulin A (IgA), which further helps to keep bad germs out and the immune system functioning properly.
3. To provide beneficial flora that help with the digestion and absorption of your food, maximizing nutrition and keeping you healthy.

Your gut contains both "good" and friendly bacteria as well as "bad" or unfriendly bacteria. The good bacteria help regulate your immune system, so it knows what is foreign and what is "you." When the balance between good and bad bacteria is disrupted, your immune system suffers. A poorly regulated immune system is more prone to autoimmunity.

Each part of the body has a different set of microbes that keep things under control. Gut microbes differ from skin microbes, which differ from microbes in your throat. Problems arise when these bugs start to grow in areas where they don't belong. For example, gut bacteria growing in your bladder will cause a urinary tract infection. Your immune system usually knows to get rid of things that aren't where they should be in order to protect the function of an organ or body part. But when your immune system is disrupted, you may develop both digestive and immune issues.

The constant communication between your gut microbes and your intestinal lining maintains a healthy immune system balance. When your immune system is in balance, your digestive tract works well, and you can break down and absorb necessary nutrients, eliminate what needs to go, and protect your body from harmful substances. The problem is that not everyone has a well-functioning gut. And as I mentioned, digestive problems are even more common in people with Lyme disease.

Lyme Disease and Gut Issues

Countless people with Lyme disease report years of poor gut health. People with active Lyme disease may experience intestinal problems such as the following:

- Chronic constipation
- Diarrhea
- Abdominal pain
- Gas
- Bloating

It's not at all uncommon for this digestive distress to turn into a more serious condition, such as Crohn's disease, inflammatory bowel disorder, or ulcerative colitis.[3] One study found that more than 25 percent of people with acute Lyme disease had other digestive issues, such as anorexia, nausea, vomiting, abdominal pain, or an enlarged spleen or liver.[4] This suggests that Lyme disease may cause these chronic gastrointestinal problems.

Inflammation and Leaky Gut

What do all these ailments have in common? Inflammation. The physiological, psychological, and toxic stressors that my plan targets can lead to both abnormal changes in intestinal microbes and inflammation. And as the intestinal lining becomes more inflamed, the protective barrier of cells that keep harmful bugs and foreign substances from entering your body begins to break down.

Imagine if a dam developed little pinholes in its concrete walls. The water would slowly start to trickle in. And if there were enough pinholes, a large amount of water would pass through the dam. It is the same in the human body. The protective barriers, such as the skin or mucous membranes, are here to keep unwanted invaders out. But if foreign microbes or food particles can easily pass through those barriers, they can stimulate your immune system, causing further inflammation. You see how this can become a vicious cycle—once your barricade has been damaged, it is hard to turn off the immune reaction and inflammation continues to get worse and worse. In the medical world, we call this intestinal hyperpermeability, but it is more commonly known as *leaky gut*. So to repair the damage, you have to plug up these holes in the dam.

HEALING LEAKY GUT

Leaky gut is exactly what it sounds like. As the protective intestinal lining breaks down, the normally tight spaces between the gut cells become loose, undermining the gut's capacity to act as a filter. Leaky gut has been associated with depression, obesity, Parkinson's disease, type 2 diabetes, Crohn's disease, ulcerative colitis, celiac disease, IBS, and trauma, as well as with long-term use of NSAIDs like ibuprofen, infection, immune suppression, radiation, and stress.[5] You will recognize that many of these are the same as the autoimmune conditions associated with Lyme disease (see Appendix C, page 334).

Diet is a major contributor to leaky gut. It has also been linked to drinking too much alcohol[6] and eating a diet high in unhealthy fats, such as lard or cottonseed oil.[7] Eating a low-fiber diet also seems to make leaky gut worse, as your normal bacteria use the fiber to replicate.[8] Having an acidic gut doesn't help either,[9] which is why in Chapter 4 I recommend following an alkaline diet.

Now that you understand the crucial role of gut health, let's get started to repair your gut and its cousin, your immune system.

The Immune-Boosting Gut Protocol

The good news is that even if you have taken antibiotics or other medications like NSAIDs that may have altered your gut flora or you have not been eating as well as you should, you can turn things around with the Immune-Boosting Gut Protocol. The protocol consists of these supports for your gut:

- Probiotics
- Glutamine
- Digestive enzymes
- Fish oil
- Resveratrol
- Herbs

Probiotics: Bring the Good Guys Back

The single best thing to help repair your gut, whether the damage was caused by dietary factors or using NSAIDS, is a good-quality probiotic.[10] What is good quality?

When I was a medical student, we sent twenty different probiotics from professional-grade to consumer companies to be analyzed for their content. To our surprise, only *one* of them actually had the exact strains of probiotics and quantity listed on the product label. An ongoing problem for many probiotics companies is being able to keep the organisms alive after they are manufactured. Use products that have been well researched for their purity and stability once they go on the shelf. Some products need to be refrigerated to keep the organisms alive. Others are stable at room temperature. Make sure to follow the manufacturer's guidelines on storage as well as on when and how to take them so that you get the best results.

Many studies show the beneficial effects of taking probiotics to rebuild a damaged gut wall.[11] Probiotics are usually measured in colony-forming units (CFU) as a way to know how many live organisms are in each capsule, tablet, or powder. It's a little misleading because, while you would think having a higher colony count is better, that is not necessarily true. Different probiotics seem to work at varying amounts, so taking a probiotic that contains 50 billion CFUs is not necessarily better than taking a different product that has only 10 billion CFUs. Studies have examined many different probiotics at various amounts and there is no clear indication that more is better—they are just different.

You will find that most of the better products are more expensive than lesser-quality products. With probiotics, you definitely get what you pay for. Although research does not show that rotating probiotics is necessary, most of my patients feel better taking two or three different probiotics and rotating them weekly.

Please choose from the following:

- *Lactobacillus rhamnosus* (Lacto GG), often sold as Culturelle, is one of the most well-researched probiotics in the world and has been shown to help modulate inflammation and repair a leaky gut.[12] Each adult capsule provides 10 billion CFUs. Take one capsule once or twice a day with food. It can be kept at room temperature.
- VSL#3 contains eight strains of beneficial bacteria. Available in either capsule or sachet, this product has been shown to help reduce inflammation that leads to leaky gut.[13] Each capsule provides 112 billion CFUs. The powder in each sachet provides 450 billion CFUs. VSL#3 is also available in prescription strength, with each sachet containing 900 billion CFUs. Take one capsule daily with food. If you prefer to take the powder, start with ½ sachet daily with food and increase up to a full sachet if tolerated. It must be refrigerated. You can purchase this product directly from the company at VSL3.com.
- Ther-Biotic Complete comprises twelve strains of bacteria. Take one capsule two times a day with food. It must be refrigerated.
- Probiotic Plus contains 100 billion CFUs. I had this formula made for my patients. These strains have all been shown to help protect the gut from infection and reduce inflammation.[14] Take one capsule daily with food. It can be kept at room temperature. This product is available through my website at dariningelsnd.com/store.

- Theralac has five probiotic strains with 30 billion CFUs. Take one capsule twice a day with food. It can be kept at room temperature.
- Prescript-Assist is a soil-based probiotic, which means it contains bacteria you would normally find in the ground. We naturally ingest these microbes when we eat various plants. Although they do not make up the majority of our normal gut flora, I have seen people with chronic bowel problems get better when using this product. At least one study found that it helped reduce abdominal pain in people with IBS.[15] It contains twenty-nine strains of bacteria and I find that it is well tolerated. Take one capsule two times a day with food. It does not need to be refrigerated.
- *Saccharomyces boulardii* is a beneficial yeast and not a bacteria like other probiotics. I use this when the most troubling symptom is loose stool or diarrhea. It can help slow things down and help your gut to heal.[16] Take two capsules two times a day if having diarrhea and then one capsule twice a day after you start having normal bowel movements.

There are many other high-quality probiotics on the market, so talk with your nutritionally oriented health-care provider or check out the Resources section (page 325) for more information on high-quality products.

Glutamine: Give Your Cells the Food They Need

The most abundant amino acid in the body is the amino acid glutamine, the main source of energy to the lining of the small intestines. As these cells get damaged from leaky gut, glutamine can help rebuild new, healthy cells. It also has immune-modulating benefits.[17] Amino acids are the building blocks of protein, but most proteins are too large to pass across the intestinal wall.

Most bodily glutamine is stored in your muscles. If you have low muscle mass, your glutamine levels may already be depleted. Several studies show that taking glutamine supplements helps maintain the integrity of the gut barrier and improve immune function.[18] Glutamine is always part of my gut-rebuilding program for those with leaky gut but should be avoided for those with inflammatory bowel disease such as ulcerative colitis or Crohn's disease, as well as those with poor liver function, as glutamine supplementation can make these conditions worse.

Start with 1,000 milligrams twice a day before meals. This is a small dose to make sure you tolerate it well. You can continue to increase the dose by 1,000 milligrams daily, up to 15 grams per day. While this may sound like a high amount to take, the research shows that people require high doses to help heal the gut. You should take 15 grams daily only with medical supervision. Doses up to 40 grams a day have been used safely, but higher amounts can cause abdominal pain or loose stool in some people and should therefore be used carefully.

Enzymes: Aid to Digestion

The standard American diet (SAD) is unfortunately filled with many highly processed and genetically modified foods, which your body may not be able to break down. The digestive system takes large proteins, carbohydrates, and fats and breaks them into small bits that can be absorbed in the small intestine easily. However, if the digestive process doesn't work well, partially digested molecules can proceed through the digestive tract. The immune system may not recognize them. In the effort to eliminate these unknown substances, the immune system tries to attack them, creating more inflammation.

Digestion begins in the mouth, where enzymes in saliva start breaking down carbohydrates and protein. Food then moves into the stomach, which releases hydrochloric acid to digest proteins. Once food leaves the stomach, it enters the small intestine (duodenum), where pancreatic and gallbladder enzymes continue the process of breaking down the rest of your food. Most nutrients get absorbed in the first part of the small intestine, the location for a lot of digestive activity. Digestive enzymes help maintain the intestinal wall to keep bad microbes out.[19] Taking digestive enzymes can help strengthen the intestine by reducing symptoms of gas, bloating, belching, heartburn, and diarrhea.

Choose one among these digestive enzyme products:

- Vital-Zymes Complete contains enzymes to aid in digesting proteins, carbohydrates, and fat. There is also a children's version of this product that is chewable. Take one capsule or chewable tablet with each full meal.
- Dipan-9 contains pancreatin, which is a combination of amylase, lipase, and protease. It is especially good if you have a difficult time eating fatty foods and feel that you don't digest them well. Take one capsule with each full meal.
- Enzalase has twelve different enzymes to help break down your food and stimulate growth of your healthy bacteria. Take one capsule with each full meal.

Digestive enzymes are generally very well tolerated, even if you have a sensitive stomach. You might notice some gas or bloating for the first few days of taking digestive enzymes, but this should pass quickly as your digestion improves. You should not take digestive enzymes if you have an active stomach ulcer or any disease of the pancreas.

Fish Oil: An Excellent Source of Omega-3 Fatty Acids

Fish oil has a large amount of omega-3 fatty acids, which do many good things for your body, including decreasing your blood pressure, reducing your cholesterol, improving your memory, lifting your mood, making your skin soft, and strengthening your gut barrier.[20] The fatty acids in fish oil that confer these benefits are eicosapentaenoic acid (EPA) and docosahexaenoic acid (DHA). EPA is a natural anti-inflammatory as well and can help reduce your joint and muscle pain.

Research shows that taking fish oil in combination with probiotics enhances the intestinal cell lining, making it stronger.[21] Other studies have found similar results.[22] Most studies have used either fish oil (salmon or sardines, for example) or cod liver oil, but krill oil is a great option if you have difficulty swallowing capsules, since you can usually get an equal amount of EPA and DHA in a smaller capsule of krill oil. Krill oil is effective at reducing inflammation and protecting the gut wall.[23]

Note that cod liver oil naturally contains high amounts of vitamin A and vitamin D. If you have liver disease, it's inadvisable to take fish or krill oil for an extended period of time. I recommend 3,000 milligrams a day divided into two doses and taken with food. If you take fish oil on an empty stomach, it might repeat on you. Use capsules or liquids—whichever is easier for you. If you get a liquid, make sure to keep it in the refrigerator, as fish oil becomes rancid quickly.

Liquid fish oil can deliver more omega-3 fatty acids per dose than capsules, but if you don't like the taste of liquid fish oil, capsules are a good option. Some of the products I recommend include the following:

- Carlson Cod Liver Oil (lemon flavored): Adults take one tablespoon daily with food; children take one teaspoon two times a day with food.
- Nordic Naturals ProOmega: Take two capsules three times a day with food.
- Krill oil: I have my own brand or you can use Thorne Research brand. Take two capsules twice a day with food.
- Super Omega: This highly concentrated monoglyceride fish oil is designed to have up to three times greater absorption of DHA and EPA than other fish oil products. Take two capsules twice a day with food. This can be found in my store at dariningelsnd.com/store.

If you are a vegetarian or vegan, you can use flaxseed oil instead of fish oil. Flaxseed oil is also high in omega-3 fatty acids, but mostly in the form of alpha-linolenic acid (ALA), which needs to be converted into EPA and DHA in order for your body to use it. Although it may take a little more work for the body to make EPA and DHA from flaxseed oil, studies show that it is also useful in repairing leaky gut.[24]

Chemicals in conventional flaxseed products can add to your toxic load. Look instead for organic flaxseed oil products such as the following:

- Barlean's Organic Flax Oil: Take one tablespoon daily with food.
- Barlean's Organic Flax Oil Capsules: Take three capsules twice a day with food.

You can also increase your consumption of omega-3 fat-containing foods. Unfortunately, many fresh fish are contaminated with lead and mercury, while farm-raised fish are often high in polychlorinated bi-phenyls (PCBs). Make sure to stick with fish that are low in contami-nants, such as the following:

- Wild salmon
- Sole
- Perch
- Pike
- Whitefish (haddock, pollock, cod)
- Red snapper
- Ocean trout
- Sardines

Avoid game fish, such as tuna, grouper, shark, marlin, swordfish, and Chilean sea bass, as they are higher in toxic metals. Try to eat some healthy fish two to three times per week. If you are vegan, try to eat at least four servings a day of nuts and seeds to get these benefi-cial fats.

Resveratrol: Nature's Antioxidant

Found in the skin of red grapes (and lesser amounts in peanuts and berries), resveratrol belongs to a class of compounds called polyphe-nols. These help reduce inflammation, protect against heart disease and cancer, regulate blood sugar, and improve memory.[25] In France, where people regularly drink red wine, the incidence of heart disease is much lower than in other Western countries, despite the French love of rich foods. The resveratrol in wine may account for this phenomenon, which is known as *the French paradox*.

Resveratrol can stop gut inflammation and protect the intestinal barrier.[26] It can mildly stop the Lyme organism from reproducing.[27] It has also been shown to help with several neurological diseases, such as Alzheimer's and Parkinson's disease.[28] Although there are no specific studies showing that resveratrol prevents or reverses memory loss or cognitive impairment in Lyme disease, given the similarity of these other illnesses, it may be worthwhile to take it.

While drinking moderate amounts of red wine can definitely help you get resveratrol, most people with Lyme disease do not handle alcohol very well, even in small quantities. Instead, take a supplement that contains 250 milligrams per capsule. Take one capsule twice a day. If you have poor memory or neuropathy (numbness or tingling in your hands, feet, or skin), take two capsules twice a day.

Other Herbs to Heal Leaky Gut

Although there is no research on most herbs recommended to heal leaky gut, there is a long tradition of using certain plants. If you like drinking tea, you'll love taking either slippery elm (*Ulmus fulva*) or marshmallow (*Althea officinalis*). Both of these herbs are called demulcents, which means they have substances in them to soothe your stomach and intestinal lining. While most teas are served hot, slippery elm and marshmallow are best served cold. To make them, put 1 teaspoon of powder from either herb in 12 ounces of water. Mix and refrigerate overnight. The next day, you will have a thick, goopy tea. Both herbs are rich in mucilage, which gives them their characteristic texture. While it may sound and look odd, it is actually very pleasant tasting and can really make your belly feel better. Drink 12 ounces of either tea daily.

Colon Hydrotherapy to Detoxify Your Gut

As important as it is to repair your gut lining and replenish your healthy flora, it is equally important to aid your detoxification pathways, which help get rid of toxins that make you sick. One of the oldest and best ways to do this is by getting colon hydrotherapy treatments (more commonly referred to as *colonics*). The treatment involves inserting a small speculum into the rectum and gently filling the colon with warm water and then draining the contents when it's full. This process is repeated several times over the course of thirty to sixty minutes.

When I mention this to most of my patients, I often get a very strange look. Although colon hydrotherapy is not popular in the United States, it has been part of maintaining good health in many parts of Europe for decades. It may sound intimidating or even scary, but the process is actually very gentle and most people find the treatment relaxing. In addition to cleaning the colon of toxic waste, colonics also stimulate the nerves. Since the entire gastrointestinal tract (including the liver and gallbladder) is connected by the vagus nerve, this helps to eliminate toxins. The vagus nerve is the main nerve coming from your brain that helps your body relax, so stimulating this nerve promotes better digestion and elimination.

People report marked improvement after doing even just one or two colon hydrotherapy sessions. This therapy is especially helpful for chronic gas, bloating, constipation, or abdominal pain. Colon hydrotherapy is relatively safe. The single-use tube is discarded after each treatment (and the water moves in only one direction), so there is no risk of getting an infection from a previous user.

I recommend starting with treatments once or twice a week for at least three weeks. Depending on how you feel, you may continue them for longer. I have heard some people worry about washing out their good bacteria, but your gut has trillions of organisms, so losing a few million is a drop in the bucket—not to mention that bacteria replicate about every twenty minutes, so you will have replenished what was lost in a few short hours. Colon hydrotherapy is not appropriate for everyone and should be avoided if you are pregnant, or if you have rectal bleeding, colon cancer, heart disease, uncontrolled high blood pressure, or seizures.

Starting Your Path to Health

In following the Immune-Boosting Gut Protocol, you are calming inflammation, restoring the right balance between good and bad bacteria, and rebuilding a healthy immune system. But it's also essential that your diet calms inflammation and rebuilds immunity, rather than continuing the damage to your immune system. In Chapter 4, I will show you which foods are best for you and which ones you should avoid. You will learn how the Immune-Boosting Diet will alkalinize your body and strengthen and balance your immune system as you heal from Lyme disease. Even if you don't have Lyme or aren't sure if you do, you can use this diet to reduce your risk.

CHAPTER 4

The Lyme Solution Immune-Boosting Diet

While no one yet is doing the kind of research that proves that having a strong and stable immune system can prevent Lyme, at the very least, there is no harm in strengthening your immunity. In the best-case scenario, it can fortify your health. Even if there is no need for you to treat an active case of Lyme disease, you can decrease your risk factors by preventively undertaking the diet in this chapter.

In Chapter 3, you read about the connection between immunity and the gut. You learned why immune health starts with gut health. You learned how the wrong foods and diet can adversely affect your gut. But what diet will really help build a healthy gut, restore a balanced immune system, and, most important, help you recover from Lyme disease?

Which Diet Is Best for Healing Lyme Disease?

If you follow popular media, you've read about various diets that offer quick fixes for whatever ailments bother you. The problem with these—and most diets—is that they don't take into account the specific causes of *your* health condition. As a result, they don't address the real root of the problem. This often leaves people with Lyme disease trying diet after diet and finding that none of them makes a difference.

As you learned in Chapter 2, the primary underlying conditions *The Lyme Solution* will address are the troubled immune system and the gut symptoms that result. So what does an *effective* diet look like? To target the specific problems that people fighting Lyme disease require, let's step back and look at what Lyme disease is and what it does.

Symptom: Lyme disease causes persistent inflammation—in the form of joint pain, headaches, muscle aches, brain fog, abdominal pain, and other symptoms. *Takeaway:* An Immune-Boosting Diet must address inflammation.

Symptom: Food sensitivities (and allergies) often trigger immune system reactions. *Takeaway:* An Immune-Boosting Diet must reduce or eliminate the most common triggers for sensitivities and allergies.

With these takeaways in mind, over the last two decades, I put the people who came to see me on a wide range of food regimens. The diets all had their adherents, and many are beneficial for other conditions. But I was puzzled that they did not work that well for people with Lyme disease, too. When I began using the Immune-Boosting Diet, I discovered what was missing from these other nutritional approaches.

The Immune-Boosting Diet

Making dietary changes is never easy, but when you try it and start feeling better, you'll realize it's worth the effort. The diet is designed so that you eat the foods that optimize your alkalinity and avoid foods that make you more acidic. The two-week meal plan and a few dozen great recipes, offered at the end of the book, help make this as easy as possible for you. Check out the food lists in this chapter and stock your refrigerator with the delicious foods I recommend that help increase alkalinity. If you are like most people, changing your diet can be perplexing at first. Go slowly if you need to. In the following section you will find some great tips for making the transition into an alkaline diet, so be patient with the process and join us on my website (dariningelsnd.com) for extra help with diet, recipes, and other nutritional information.

Remember, this is a process—the diet can take some time to fully incorporate into your daily life. But the sooner you can implement these changes, the sooner you will start to feel better.

. . . .

Five Tips to Make Your Diet Work

1. Don't feel pressured to change everything at once. You've spent years developing your dietary habits and they won't necessarily change overnight. Start by changing just two to three foods in your diet every few days. Soon you will find yourself eating a healthier, alkaline diet.
2. Work with a professional. If you get overwhelmed, then I recommend finding a nutritionist who can help you with shopping, meal planning, and even food preparation. Sometimes a little hand-holding in the beginning can get you going on the right path to managing your diet.
3. Don't reinvent the wheel. It's great to reach out to a local support group or online forum where people share their recipe ideas as well as what worked for them. The Internet has become an invaluable resource for great recipes for nutritious, tasty meals.
4. Cook simple. You may feel like you need to make complicated or extravagant recipes, but you can keep it simple in the kitchen by using just a few ingredients. One of my favorite dishes is roasted beets, with celery and capers with a little apple cider vinegar. Find easy-to-prepare dishes that you enjoy eating.

5. Plan ahead. When you are tired and feeling unwell, it's an extra challenge to remember to buy the right foods. People who don't cook much often find shopping daunting. To make shopping easier, sit down before you go to the store to make a detailed list of what you plan to purchase.

. . . .

Diet Basics

To begin, follow a regular meal pattern and eat at least three times per day. If you are prone to low blood sugar, eat between-meal snacks. Although you are not counting calories, keep in mind that most adults need between 1,800 and 2,500 calories per day. Children need between 1,200 and 2,000 calories per day. This amount can be adjusted for age, gender, and activity level. A wearable health-tracking device can help you measure your activity level to see if you need to adjust your calorie intake. Men generally need more calories than women, and active people need more calories than sedentary people. If you want to lose weight, you can elect to reduce food intake to 1,500 calories per day. It also helps to combine the diet with a regular exercise regimen.

Meal Plans for the Two-Week Diet

The meal plans for the two-week diet are based on the do's and don'ts you've just read. Following this carefully thought-out meal plan will provide you with fourteen days of delicious and nourishing meals that will support your detoxification. Feel free to modify and adapt these suggestions, while staying within the basic guidelines.

DAY 1	
Breakfast	Warm Buckwheat Bowl
Midmorning Snack	Turmeric and Garlic Hummus with crudités
Lunch	Anti-Inflammatory Butternut Squash Stew
Midafternoon Snack	Super-Seed Crackers with Pomegranate and Avocado Salsa
Dinner	Citrus, Red Onion, and Coconut Chicken with Cast-Iron Roasted Sunchokes and Burdock Root
DAY 2	
Breakfast	Morning Boost Smoothie
Midmorning Snack	Fatigue-Fighting Green Thyme Tea
Lunch	Chicken, Greens, and Quinoa Salad with Flu-Fighter Immune Fries
Midafternoon Snack	Simple Vegetable Broth
Dinner	Roasted vegetables with Roasted Garlic Sauce and Marinade
DAY 3	
Breakfast	Simple Detox Smoothie
Midmorning Snack	Organic apple with almond butter
Lunch	Ingels's Lentil Soup and Arugula, Beet, and Super-Seed Salad with Citrus Green Tahini Dressing
Midafternoon Snack	Cassava and Multi-Seed Flatbread with almond butter
Dinner	Curried Turkey Breast with Okra

DAY 4	
Breakfast	Overnight Vanilla Oats and Chia
Midmorning Snack	Berries with Vanilla-Coconut Whipped Cream
Lunch	Quick Immune-Soothing Bone Broth and lentil burger with Spicy Cabbage Slaw
Midafternoon Snack	Chipotle Avocado Mash
Dinner	Vegan Zucchini Lasagna
DAY 5	
Breakfast	Delightful Detox Smoothie Bowl
Midmorning Snack	Coconut Yogurt Parfait
Lunch	Healthy Gut Kimchi Roll and Detox Salad
Midafternoon Snack	Ultimate Immune Lollipop
Dinner	Braised wild-caught salmon and roasted cauliflower with Crunchy Marinated Kale Salad
DAY 6	
Breakfast	Scrambled eggs with gluten-free tortilla
Midmorning Snack	Chia Pudding Deluxe with Mango
Lunch	Carrot, Ginger, and Squash Soup, gluten-free bread and Chickpea, Avocado, and Baby Tomato Salad
Midafternoon Snack	Brussels Sprout Chips
Dinner	Maitake Mushroom and Cauliflower Stir-Fry with Hijiki Seaweed Salad

DAY 7	
Breakfast	Smoked salmon on a gluten-free bagel with dairy-free cream cheese
Midmorning Snack	Hydrating Watermelon, Pear, and Mint Drink
Lunch	Lentil burger with Lemon-Sesame Green Beans
Midafternoon Snack	Vanilla-Almond Immune Shake
Dinner	Kale, Turkey, and Butternut Squash Bowl with Mashed-Up Veggie Delight
DAY 8	
Breakfast	Overnight Vanilla Oats and Chia
Midmorning Snack	Fatigue-Fighting Green Thyme Tea with Super-Seed Crackers
Lunch	Broccoli–bok choy stir-fry with Thai almond dressing
Midafternoon Snack	Celery sticks with hard-boiled egg
Dinner	Turkey cauliflower curry with mashed sweet potato
DAY 9	
Breakfast	Simple Detox Smoothie
Midmorning Snack	Black bean hummus with cucumber slices
Lunch	Lentil burger with spinach salad
Midafternoon Snack	Quick Immune-Soothing Bone Broth with scallions
Dinner	Braised wild-caught salmon with asparagus and dill rice

DAY 10	
Breakfast	Warm Buckwheat Bowl with blueberries
Midmorning Snack	Organic pear with almond butter
Lunch	Baked lentil loaf and Arugula, Beet, and Super-Seed Salad with Citrus Green Tahini Dressing
Midafternoon Snack	Coconut Yogurt Parfait
Dinner	Mini-meatballs with zucchini pasta with pesto sauce
DAY 11	
Breakfast	Morning Boost Smoothie
Midmorning Snack	Cassava and Multi-Seed Flatbread with almond butter
Lunch	Chicken, Walnut, and Apple Salad over mixed greens with lemon-oil dressing
Midafternoon Snack	Ultimate Immune Lollipop
Dinner	Harvest Vegetable Stew with chickpeas
DAY 12	
Breakfast	Eggs over easy with fried quinoa patties
Midmorning Snack	Berries with Vanilla-Coconut Whipped Cream
Lunch	Open-faced nut butter and cucumber-sprouts and avocado sandwich on gluten-free bread
Midafternoon Snack	Turmeric and Garlic Hummus with carrot sticks
Dinner	Turkey burger with Crunchy Marinated Kale Salad

DAY 13	
Breakfast	Smoked salmon on a gluten-free bagel with dairy-free cream cheese
Midmorning Snack	Vanilla-Almond Immune Shake
Lunch	Healthy Gut Kimchi Roll and Detox Salad
Midafternoon Snack	Kale chips with Garlic Flax Mayo
Dinner	Vegan Zucchini Lasagna
DAY 14	
Breakfast	Scrambled eggs with gluten-free tortilla
Midmorning Snack	Hydrating Watermelon, Pear, and Mint Drink
Lunch	Asian chicken wings with Lemon-Sesame Green Beans
Midafternoon Snack	Chia Pudding Deluxe with raspberries
Dinner	Sesame broccoli-zucchini stir-fry with Hijiki Seaweed Salad

What You Can and Cannot Eat

Notice that there are three categories of foods:

1. Generously consumed foods: Very alkaline to low-alkaline foods should make up 80 percent of your diet. Pick foods in this category and eat until satiated.
2. Modestly consumed foods: These foods are low-acid-forming foods.
3. Limited or eliminated foods: Some foods are too acidic to be part of your recovery, so you will be omitting the foods on this list as much as possible.

EAT ALL YOU WANT
(VERY TO LOW ALKALINE-FORMING)

VEGETABLES

Artichokes

Asparagus

Beets, beet greens

Broccoli

Brussels sprouts

Cabbage

Carrots

Cauliflower

Celery

Chard

Collard greens

Cucumbers

Endive

Garlic

Green beans

Jerusalem artichokes
   (sunchokes)

Kale

Kelp

Lettuces

Mustard greens

Okra

Onions

Parsley

Parsnips

Peas

Radishes

Rutabaga

Scallions

Seaweeds (nori, dulse, etc.)

Spinach

Sprouted grains

Sprouts

Squash

Sweet potato

Turnips

Watercress

Yams

Zucchini

FRUITS

Bananas

Pomegranates

Raisins

Watermelon

NUTS/SEEDS/NUT BUTTERS

Almonds

Cashews

Chia

Coconut

Flaxseeds

Pumpkin seeds

Sesame seeds

Sunflower seeds

GRAINS/LEGUMES

Amaranth

Buckwheat

Kamut

Lentils

Lima beans

Millet

Mung beans

Navy beans

Pinto beans

Red beans

Quinoa

Spelt

White beans

OILS

Organic avocado oil

Organic coconut oil

Organic extra-virgin, cold-
    pressed olive oil

Organic flaxseed oil

Organic safflower oil

* Note that most oils use solvents in
their extraction process, so buying
organic oils will help keep you from
consuming toxic chemicals.

BEVERAGES

Alkaline water

Green drinks (kale, celery,
    cucumber, parsley, lime,
    cilantro, chard, collards,
    spinach)

Herbal teas (decaffeinated)

Water (tap, spring, mineral)

EAT NO MORE THAN 1 CUP OR WHOLE PIECE A DAY

VEGETABLES

Eggplant

Peppers

Tomatoes

White potato

FRUITS
Avocado
Grapefruit
Grapes
Lemon
Lime

EAT NO MORE THAN FIVE TIMES PER WEEK
(MILDLY ACID-FORMING)

MEAT AND EGGS
Beef
Chicken
Eggs
Pork
Turkey

FRUITS
Apples
Apricots
Berries
Cantaloupe
Cherries
Honeydew melon
Mango
Nectarines
Oranges
Papaya
Peaches
Pineapple
Plums
Tangerines

NUTS/SEEDS
Pecans
Pine nuts

GRAINS/LEGUMES
Brown rice
Hemp
Oats
Rye
Soy products, except soy sauce
    (organic only)
Wheat (organic only)
White rice

FISH/SHELLFISH (WILD ONLY)
Mackerel
Perch
Pike
Roughy
Salmon
Sardines

Shellfish (shrimp, lobster, clams, mussels, etc.)

Sole

Tilapia

OILS

Organic grapeseed oil

Organic hempseed oil

Organic sunflower oil

SWEETENERS

Coconut sugar

Lo-han

Stevia

FOODS TO AVOID WHILE ON THE PROGRAM

FARM-RAISED FISH

Farm-raised fish may be high in polychlorinated biphenyls (PCBs) and other toxic chemicals, which are known carcinogens.

DAIRY PRODUCTS

Butter

Cheese

Ice cream

Milk

Sour cream

Yogurt

DRIED FRUITS

Except raisins

NUTS/SEEDS

Brazil nuts

Hazelnuts

Macadamia nuts

Peanuts

Pistachios

Walnuts

ADDITIVES, ARTIFICIAL DYES, FLAVORINGS, SWEETENERS, AND PRESERVATIVES

All nitrates, nitrites, and sulfites (used as preservatives)

Aluminum

Aspartame

Carrageenan

Ethylparaben

Formaldehyde

Methylparaben

Monosodium glutamate (MSG)

Propylene glycol

Saccharin

Sodium benzoate or benzoic acid

Sucralose

Tartrazine (yellow #5) and other
    artificial dyes

Canned foods (containing lots of
    preservatives and chemicals)

Corn and all corn derivatives
    (contained in most processed
    foods in the United States)

Corn starch

Corn syrup

Dextrin

Fructose

Glucose

High-fructose corn syrup

Maltodextrin

Sorbitol

JUNK SNACK FOODS

Cake

Candy

Chips

Chocolate/cocoa

Cookies

Cupcakes

Doughnuts

Pastries

Pies

Popcorn

Processed food

Processed or refined crackers

SWEETENERS

Agave syrup

Honey

Sugar (white and brown)

YEAST

Beer

Breads

Red wine

CONDIMENTS

Jam

Jelly

Margarine

Mustard

Soy sauce

White vinegar (made from corn)

OILS

All hydrogenated oils and trans
    fats, including shortening,
    margarine, cottonseed oil,
    peanut oil, and corn oil

Corn oil

Cottonseed oil

Soybean oil

Vegetable oil

BEVERAGES

Alcohol

Black tea

Coffee

Fruit juice

Soda

Sports drinks

How Is the Immune-Boosting Diet Different from Other Diets?

You might think that my diet sounds like a lot of other diets, so let me explain why it's different. First, let's look at what most people are actually eating.

When people first come into my office, the majority are eating a standard American diet (SAD). High in simple carbs and filled with junk food and soda, the most common American diet contains highly processed foods and few vegetables. It offers little to no fiber and is low on fluid intake. Eating such a diet over many years alters the internal environment of your gut—and not in a good way. Your gut cells don't function optimally. Acids build up in your body, leading to fatigue, inflammation in the muscles and joints, allergies, poor brain and intestinal function, headaches, and sleep disturbances.

How does this happen? When gut bacteria break down your food, acid is one of the by-products. If, like many people, you eat a SAD diet and have developed gut flora imbalances, those acid by-products of digestion may be excessive or abnormal. While all the complex mechanisms are not fully understood, some researchers suggest that an overly acidic dietary pH leaves people with mildly elevated acid levels. When this *metabolic acidosis* persists over time, it alters kidney and gut function.

Almost any healthy diet is better than the SAD diet, which so radically undermines function. But diets that work for other conditions may not work for people with Lyme disease, because they do not alter your body's pH levels. When a diet increases bodily alkalinity and decreases acidity, it supports immune system health. I will explore the reasons for this more thoroughly later on in this chapter. But first let's take a look at the most commonly proposed diets for Lyme treatment.

The Paleo Diet

Perhaps the most popular diet many people with Lyme disease follow is the high-protein, low-carbohydrate paleo diet. This diet supports weight loss and helps to prevent or relieve conditions such as diabetes, high blood pressure, high cholesterol, and heart disease. The low carb intake helps regulate blood sugar and many of the hormones involved with metabolism. The paleo diet also involves eating less refined and processed food. In fact, many of its health benefits can be attributed to better-quality food.

But despite its many benefits, the paleo diet has one downside for people with Lyme disease that I will unfold a bit later on in this section on nutrition for Lyme.

The Anti-Candida Diet

Many people believe that the well-known anti-Candida diet can be helpful for Lyme disease. In case you are not aware of it, this diet was popularized in the 1980s by Dr. William Crook, author of *The Yeast Connection.* Crook recognized that yeast overgrowth in the body was linked to fatigue, joint pain, brain fog, and other health conditions. Since then, there have been several versions of the anti-Candida diet. The common theme of these diets is to restrict all sources of sugar, whether from natural sources or not, including alcohol, soda, fruit, grains, beans, and artificial food additives. The goal of restricting sugar, or simple carbohydrates, as nutritionists call them, is to selectively starve the yeasts that normally live in our body in order to keep them from overgrowing and causing adverse health problems. Some people believe that if this diet can starve the yeast, it may also "starve" Lyme and other microbes that are out of control.

Other Popular Diets

The Zone Diet, South Beach Diet, Atkins Diet, and Blood Type Diet are designed to help encourage weight loss and improve cardiovascular and overall health but are not specific to any one condition. The Specific Carbohydrate Diet (SCD) is used to treat inflammatory bowel disease. All of these diets drastically reduce simple carbohydrate intake, because it is clear that there are many health benefits to eating less sugar and junk food.

The Benefits of pH Balancing

What is missing from all the diets I've surveyed here? First, none offer the complete range of crucial nutrients. Second, none specifically address maintaining a balanced pH. Why does that matter? Having a more-alkaline (basic) pH is an invaluable but underutilized way to reduce inflammation, rebuild the gut, and boost the immune system.

More than fourteen years ago, I made a surprising discovery. I began to experiment with a pH-balancing diet and soon discovered that it made a huge difference for those with Lyme disease. To my great surprise, it helped people turn a corner in the unrelenting process of their illness. From all that I saw clinically, I also became convinced that following this diet can help rebuild the immune system and make people more immune to Lyme disease. Over the years, I've used this diet with thousands of people and found that most people with Lyme disease improve when they eat foods that promote alkalinity. Using this approach restores optimal gut health and reduces inflammation. Like most things in life, diet is all about balance.

WHAT IS PH AND HOW DOES THE PH IN FOODS AFFECT ME?

Potential of hydrogen, or *pH*, describes how acidic or alkaline something is. On a scale from 1 to 14, a pH of 1 is highly acidic and a pH of 14 is highly alkaline. A neutral pH is 7, neither acid nor alkaline. With the exception of water, every food is on the acid/alkaline spectrum. Foods are classified as alkaline if they are high in sodium, potassium, or calcium. Foods that have more sulfur, phosphate, or chloride are considered acidic. The following table shows some foods in each category.

HIGHLY ACIDIC FOODS	MILDLY ACIDIC FOODS	SLIGHTLY ALKALINE FOODS	MOST-ALKALINE FOODS
Alcohol	Apples	Artichokes	Avocado
Artificial sweeteners	Dates	Asparagus	Broccoli
Cocoa	Eggs	Bananas	Cabbage
Coffee	Most fish	Beets	Carrots
Corn	Most meats (including beef, chicken, and pork)	Blueberries	Chard
Dairy products		Brussels sprouts	Kale
Dried fruits (except raisins)	Oats	Cauliflower	Lemons
		Celery	Lentils
			Limes

HIGHLY ACIDIC FOODS	MILDLY ACIDIC FOODS	SLIGHTLY ALKALINE FOODS	MOST-ALKALINE FOODS
Jam/jelly	Plums	Cucumbers	Nectarines
Peanuts	Rice	Grapes	Onions
Soda	Rye	Green beans	Parsley
Yeast	Soy	Lettuce	Pineapple
	Wheat	Oranges	Raspberries
		Peas	Seaweed
		Strawberries	Spinach
			Sweet potato
			Watermelon
			Zucchini

The pH noted in the preceding table represents how foods influence body pH *after* they are digested and assimilated. For example, lemons are very acidic but promote alkaline formation after you eat them. It is this result—how the food ultimately affects the body—that this chart reveals.

Why Does pH Matter?

The goal of the Immune-Boosting Diet is to restore and maintain a healthy body pH. When the body maintains a healthy pH, all of its cells function as nature intended.

To comprehend how this works, it helps to know that each tissue, organ, and fluid in the body has an optimal pH at which the cells and enzymes work best. If in any bodily location the pH starts to become too acidic or too alkaline, then normal function stops or slows down, leading to future disease. The complex interaction between our cells, nervous system, and hormones ensures that each tissue, organ, and fluid works at an optimal pH level. Changes in one bodily area may lead to changes in another. Therefore, changing pH in the gut can lead to changes in pH in other organs and tissues. For example, alterations in gut pH can affect the gut flora's production of short-chain fatty acids, which are crucial for energy metabolism.[1] If the gut pH isn't balanced correctly, the downstream result is less energy and more fatigue. And this is just one area of function.

Let's look at another: the stomach pH is highly acidic (pH 1.0 to 3.5), since the acid is necessary to break down complex proteins into its smaller chain amino acids, making them easier to absorb in the small intestine. By contrast, the pH of the first part of the small intestine is alkaline (pH 7.0 to 8.5), to help neutralize the acid it receives from the stomach. The pH of the blood ranges from 7.35 to 7.45, slightly alkaline. (Blood pH is tightly regulated, independently of the pH of your food. The Immune-Boosting Diet does not change blood pH, nor is it intended to.)

ORGAN	NORMAL PH
Skin	4.0 to 6.5
Stomach	1.35 to 3.5
Bile	7.6 to 8.8
Urine	6.8 to 8.0
Cerebrospinal fluid	7.3
Blood	7.35 to 7.45

Keeping the body in a more-alkaline state is a heightened challenge for the stressed immune systems of people with Lyme disease for four main reasons:

1. The immune system may have already been compromised prior to receiving a tick bite.
2. The immune system is undermined both by Lyme disease and by the standard medical treatments of Lyme disease.

3. Obtaining healthy nutrition takes special effort in the current food environment, where cheap, unhealthy, and nutritionally depleted foods are the norm.
4. The earth itself is progressively becoming more acidic.

When so many diverse external factors—an insect bite, a medical treatment with side effects, an unhealthy food system, and ecological acidification—all challenge your immunity at once, it's not surprising for health to suffer. But alkalinizing your diet can truly help. For starters, you can get a baseline and see how acid versus alkaline you are right now by taking this simple test.

. . . .

Urine Testing for pH

No test can measure tissue pH directly. Nevertheless, testing the pH of your urine can help you track your progress starting today, as you begin the program, and throughout the time you follow it. Over time, this diet will help put your body into a more-alkaline state. The aim is a urine pH of 7.3 or higher (usually, it will range from 6.8 to 8.0).

Purchase pH strips from your local pharmacy, or order them online. The strips should have a range of 1 to 14. I recommend testing your first morning urine and then testing again thirty to sixty minutes after each meal for the first two weeks of the diet.

Please keep a log of your results. The pH of your first morning urine will always be more acidic (lower), since your urine has concentrated over the night and you have not eaten anything. Once you are consistently getting alkaline pH readings, you don't need to check as often. When you feel confident that your pH is consistently alkaline, I recommend checking first thing in the morning and after dinner to make sure you are still on track. Remember, you are checking only urine pH, but this is the most accurate way to know that you're moving in the right direction.

. . . .

The Role of pH in Nature

All living creatures, including plants and animals, must maintain a healthy pH to survive. Even though slight changes in pH are often benign, such changes will affect people with pre-existing health compromises, such as poor kidney or liver function.

Let's see what happens. As the earth becomes progressively more acidic, it inevitably follows that the foods that grow on earth become more acidic and that therefore humans consume more-acidic food products. These ultimately make our own bodies more acidic. The acid environment in the natural world also affects the mineral content of foods, since growth of most plants is inhibited by acidic soil and aluminum toxicity, leading to fewer minerals being absorbed by the plants' roots.[2] Imbalances of sodium, potassium, calcium, magnesium, zinc, copper, and iron can lead to multiple problems, including hormone disruption, anemia, fatigue, muscle weakness, and an underactive thyroid, to name a few. While it may seem that small changes in pH do not matter much, the impact on human health is ongoing and builds.

Over the past hundred years, the oceans and our soil have also become increasingly acidic. These somewhat minor changes in pH destroy our natural ecosystem. For example, increased amounts of acid rain can leach aluminum from clay into rivers, lakes, and streams. This in turn can kill fish, plants, or other animals that ingest the contaminated water. When the soil becomes too acidic, certain plants can no longer grow. Any living creature that depends on that plant for survival will suffer. Highly acidic soil has also been identified as a major contributor to erosion.

Humans are also a species in the natural world, and these significant changes in our habitat all ultimately affect human health. Even if you consume a diverse and otherwise healthy diet, without taking additional nutritional supplements, it's extremely likely that you lack the right quantities of the right nutrients and the right minerals. These global changes in your environment, your food supply, and even the water you drink significantly alter nutrient levels and pH balance.

Restoring pH Balance Through the Immune-Boosting Diet

Obviously, as these global changes persist, like all species, humans will continue to be affected. And that makes it even more urgent now to maintain a healthy pH balance through diet—especially for those at risk of (or who already have) Lyme disease.

Although there are no specific studies on diet and Lyme disease, research has shown that a more-alkaline diet can help reverse this ongoing acidification and produce the following important health impacts:[3]

- Keep inflammation under control
- Improve detoxification pathways so you are better equipped to get rid of toxins
- Optimize healthy gut flora
- Benefit bone health
- Reduce muscle wasting
- Protect from chronic diseases, such as hypertension and stroke
- Increase growth hormone, which regulates muscle strength, energy, and fat and sugar metabolism; body composition, memory, and cognition; and possibly heart function
- Increase the uptake of magnesium in our cells; magnesium is required for enzymes to function properly and to activate vitamin D, which boosts the immune system[4]

- Improves the health of bones and teeth and regulates genes that help prevent cancer development[5]
- Protect against neurological illness, including multiple sclerosis[6]

As these many benefits reveal, a more-alkaline diet is helpful both for the specific needs of Lyme patients and for many other conditions. It's helpful for everyone in an acidifying world.

With that in mind, how do the other diets I've mentioned compare? Where do they fall in terms of pH balance?

On the paleo diet, people tend to eat a lot of meat—especially red meat. A high protein intake is encouraged, and meat happens to be a rich source of protein. Unfortunately for people with Lyme disease, the high meat intake can make the body very acidic. Other protein-rich foods often eaten on the paleo diet, such as eggs, certain nuts (see the list on page 99), and beans, can further acidify the body.

While the anti-Candida diet eliminates many acid-forming foods, it emphasizes eating meat and fish in quantities that can make your body more acidic. It also restricts some vegetables and beans that promote alkalinity (see the list on pages 96–97), including sweet potatoes, yams, and squash.

Instead, by following my alkalinizing Immune-Boosting Diet, people restore their pH balance and wind up experiencing relief and results—and so will you. Don't wait to experience its benefits. As you learn the basics of this diet, wherever you are on the Lyme spectrum, from worried that you might have the disease to having chronic Lyme symptoms, please start eating the foods I recommend right away. They will promote alkalinity in your body.

The Immune-Boosting Diet guides you toward the foods that will help restore your health. Unlike many diets that involve elimination of foods or calorie restriction, the Immune-Boosting Diet focuses on foods that are nutrient-dense and promote a healthy, alkaline state. Because the foods are so nutrient-dense, this diet is satiating and satisfying.

Allergies and the Immune-Boosting Diet

Although the food lists that I provide offer overall guidelines, with a challenged immune system, please remain mindful of your food allergies or intolerances. If you know that certain foods affect you, please avoid those foods, even if they're on the list. If a specific food is good for promoting alkalinity but you don't feel well after eating it, keep it out of your diet. If you suspect, but don't know for sure, that you have food allergies or intolerances, there are many different ways to find out.

First, try a simple at-home elimination diet. In this widely used approach, you eliminate certain common culprits and then reintroduce them one by one and watch for any reactions. While this takes a little work, it's the lowest-cost and easiest way to get an indication as to which foods might trigger a reaction.

Begin by eliminating all of the following foods for three weeks:

- Beans
- Beef
- Chicken
- Citrus
- Coffee
- Corn
- Dairy
- Eggplant
- Eggs

- Gluten
- Nuts
- Peppers
- Pork
- Soy
- Tomato
- White potato
- Wheat

This list covers most of the common food allergies or sensitivities I see in my practice. I know it will take some effort to avoid these items, but the upside is that if you are sensitive to any of these foods, you will actually feel better during the elimination phase. After three weeks, start reintroducing one food every three days. Pay attention to how you feel and keep notes on your symptoms. If they worsen, then you know that a particular food is not good for you. Keep in mind that symptoms can be physical, emotional, or mental, so feeling irritable after you reintroduce a food can be as significant as joint pain.

Continue with this process until each one of the seventeen foods you have eliminated has been added back. If you discover during this process that a specific food does not agree with you, then eliminate it for six months. You may then introduce it again to see if you tolerate it better. The whole process of the elimination diet takes ten to eleven weeks. Admittedly, it requires a lot of discipline, but it can provide you with valuable information about how food affects you.

What if you don't feel that you have the patience or discipline to do an elimination diet? Please talk with your functional medicine practitioner to find out about other available tests to help identify your food sensitivities or intolerances.

Should I Eat Organic or Nonorganic Foods?

Please eat as many organic foods as possible while on this diet—and in fact all the time, if you can manage to. Research shows that nonorganic foods have lower nutrient content than their organic counterparts. Many of the pesticides and herbicides used in modern farming deplete these foods of their nutrients, especially important minerals like selenium, zinc, and magnesium. Many of these same chemicals also disrupt your endocrine system, causing problems with thyroid and reproductive hormones like estrogen and testosterone.

Fortunately, the demand for organic food has grown so much that many large commercial retailers now carry organic foods at a reasonable price. If you're trying to keep a budget, take a look at the Environmental Working Group's (ewg.org) annual list of the Dirty Dozen, the top twelve foods with the highest pesticide content. In 2016, the most heavily pesticided foods were:

- Strawberries
- Apples
- Nectarines
- Peaches
- Celery
- Grapes
- Cherries
- Spinach
- Tomatoes
- Bell peppers
- Cherry tomatoes
- Cucumbers

Once you know the pesticide content of your most frequently eaten foods, you can decide which foods are worth the extra money for an organic purchase. Eating more organic foods will reduce the load of toxic chemicals in your body.

Eating patterns develop in childhood, so making changes to your diet can be difficult at first and may take time. Being consistent is the key. A few "cheat days" here and there may add up to stopping you from feeling your best. Most people notice improvements in their health within weeks of starting the Immune-Boosting Diet. And there is an added payoff: as you start to feel better, it becomes easier to stick to the rest of the program.

Six Tips for Making the Immune-Boosting Diet Work for You

Many diets advertise quick results in a short time, but that is not the purpose of the Immune-Boosting Diet. Rather, it was developed to help give you long-term results. Think of this as a marathon, not a sprint. Changing your diet can be challenging at first, but once you get the hang of it, you will find that your health improves and you start to feel more like your old self again. The key to success on this diet is to be persistent. Try not to get frustrated during the process. There may be times where you eat food that is not on the program. It's okay. A little slip-up here and there will not undo all of the hard work you've already put in. But the more diligent you are with the diet, the faster you will start to feel better. Here are six tips for making the diet work for you.

1. Start each morning with a slice of fresh lemon or lime squeezed into 8 ounces of water.

Drink it warm or cold. This morning beverage will help alkalinize your body first thing in the morning, giving you a good start. The lemon water also helps fill your stomach, so that you're not as hungry in the morning. You can also use it to replace your morning routine of coffee or tea. Drinking those common drinks may dispose you to being more acidic.

2. Cut down on and eventually eliminate coffee.

If you are a regular coffee drinker, cutting it out of your diet can be difficult. Caffeine withdrawal may give you a headache. For the first two weeks on the program, I recommend transitioning to half-caffeinated coffee (half regular and half decaf). You'll still enjoy your morning cup of joe while easing into your new morning routine. After two weeks, switch to decaf coffee only for another two weeks. Once you have passed through the phase of caffeine withdrawal, eliminate coffee completely. Use the same process if you drink caffeinated tea in the morning. Substitute water with lemon or lime, or herbal teas, such as chamomile, lemon balm, hibiscus, or other flavorful teas to help start your day.

3. Avoid processed foods for the first week of the plan.

To do that, first go through your cupboards, fridge, and freezer. Pull out any items that came in a box, can, or plastic container that are either microwavable or ready-to-eat, which is how most processed foods are packaged. Some foods like beans or whole-grain pasta might come in plastic packaging, but these have to be cooked before eating, so they are likely to have few or no added ingredients or preservatives in them. When you go grocery shopping, remember to buy foods from the perimeter of the store, since this is where most supermarkets keep their fresh foods such as meats, vegetables, fruits, eggs, and fish. By avoiding the center aisles, you'll automatically avoid most processed foods. If at first you are not accustomed to the taste of fresh foods, give yourself a few weeks. Most people are surprised to find that they come to prefer them, and eventually come to feel turned off by foods they were formerly addicted to. It's one tiny benchmark of recovery when your body comes to recognize what is healing.

4. Ask your favorite restaurants to modify their menu.

Changing your diet is more difficult if you eat out a lot, since many restaurants do not list their food ingredients on the menu and the waitstaff do not know what's in the food. However, many non-fast-food restaurants will cater to your dietary needs when asked. If there is a restaurant you frequent, ask if they can prepare dishes that work with this diet, so that you can enjoy the pleasure of good food while eating the right way to health.

5. Prepare a number of meals at one time.

When you're not feeling well, the last thing you want to do is prepare elaborate meals. Even when you're feeling great, if you are like most people, finding the time every day to shop, prepare, and cook meals can be difficult. The beauty of this program is that you can make simple meals that will both nourish you and keep your body more alkaline. I suggest picking one day of the week to prepare and cook most of your meals, portion them into glass containers, and reheat them as needed. Spending a few hours on the weekend doing the cooking for most of your meals is a huge time-saver. You can prepare smaller side dishes and salads quickly and easily on the days you wish to eat them, with little time and effort involved. To get one month of easy-to-prep meals, please visit dariningelsnd.com/store/prepdish.

6. Try one new food a week from the food list.

Changing your diet is a process, not something you must accomplish on day one. You are in for the long term, so go easy on yourself. For example, if you are not used to eating dark-green leafy vegetables, I recommend starting with just one of these vegetables at a time. They are easy to prepare and can be steamed, sautéed, or boiled in a matter of a few minutes. Foods like kale, chard, mustard greens, and beet greens are very nutrient-dense and high in calcium, iron, folate, vitamin A, and fiber. It's not just greens. Other great foods to introduce into your diet, if you are not used to eating them, are Brussels sprouts, asparagus, artichokes, lentils, and quinoa.

The recipes and menu plans I offer will help you prepare and enjoy foods that are new to you and figure out how to shift to this new way of eating. With this excellent foundation for your recovery, you can now start actively targeting the Lyme bug (and co-infections) through the protocols I offer in the next phase of the program.

CHAPTER 5

Prevent and Target
Active Infection

Up to this point in *The Lyme Solution* you have looked at the elusive nature of Lyme disease and why an immune-boosting approach works best. In the Lyme Disease Symptom Questionnaire (page 42) you gained some key understandings about how likely it is that you have Lyme disease. You also learned what tests are available to confirm that diagnosis. This chapter proceeds from the certainty (or near certainty) that you have an active Lyme infection—or that you have been bitten by a tick and need to start the preventive-stage program.

If you have been wondering what treatment to follow to get the infection under control, this chapter presents five detailed, specific protocols that I have used to help thousands of people with Lyme disease. But before we turn to the protocols, you first need to understand the underlying concept that all of these programs seek to address: bacterial load.

You probably don't think much about the quantities and types of bugs in your body. Bacteria and viruses are constantly present within you, from time to time making their presence known—when you come down with a cold, the flu, an ear infection, or some other ailment. In between these infections, apart from washing our hands, most of us ignore the ongoing presence of germs of one type or another. It's hard to do otherwise because they are not visible. Typically there is no way for the average person to measure them. Doctors can measure bacteria by doing a throat culture, stool culture, or skin culture or by testing other body fluids such as blood or spinal fluid. But these are medical procedures not routinely undertaken, except when your doctor suspects you have a bacterial infection and wants to know exactly what it is.

Bacterial Load

Bacterial load is the total number of bacteria in your body at a given time. Reducing your body's load of Lyme bacteria is essential to controlling Lyme disease. Why? Because the fewer Lyme bacteria you carry, the less your body will mount an immune response, and the fewer symptoms you will have. Let's say, for example, you are allergic to ragweed. When the pollen count is high, you will be more prone to hay fever symptoms, such as sneezing, watery or itchy eyes, and runny nose. The increased amount of pollen in the air triggers the symptoms. It's exactly the same with Lyme disease: when you have a high bacterial load, you will experience stronger immune reactions and more symptoms. Bring the load of Lyme bacteria down and you reduce the symptoms. That's the goal of the treatments presented in this chapter.

Can you ever eliminate the organism completely? Some animal studies have found Lyme DNA in mice months after the mice had been treated with antibiotics for many weeks. Similarly, suppose you got chicken pox as a five-year-old. Surprisingly, you can get shingles as a fifty-five-year-old from the same virus (varicella-zoster) that has been in your body for fifty years. Given the right set of circumstances, the virus becomes activated and begins to produce symptoms. The Lyme spirochete can also stay dormant in the body for months or years. But like varicella-zoster, it does not always cause symptoms, even if it remains in the body. In other words, you can have Lyme bacteria in your body but not have any expression of the Lyme disease. Ultimately, the state of your immune system determines whether you get Lyme disease under control such that the immune system ceases attacking your own tissues. And the first step is to limit the growth of the organism.

JULIE'S STORY

When I first met Julie, she was always tired, her hands were swollen and achy, and she complained of pain in her neck, shoulders, and arms. Her eyes twitched throughout the day and she felt worse after exercise. Her primary-care doctor had found that her thyroid was underactive, but even after taking medication for a few months, she didn't feel much better. When a functional medicine doctor started her on an anti-inflammatory diet and nutritional supplements, she felt a little better. When a test for Lyme disease came back positive, the doctor referred Julie to me.

I started her on a protocol of Chinese herbs (you will learn about these later in the chapter) to start killing the Lyme organism and reduce her inflammation. She also took an enzyme formula to increase the herbs' effectiveness at reducing the load on her body. I added an arginine formula to improve her circulation and N-acetylcysteine (NAC) to increase her glutathione levels, which are often low in those with Lyme.

Shortly thereafter, Julie emailed me that her shoulder and neck pain were almost completely gone, her energy was returning, and her hands were less swollen. We continued our work together by refining her diet in order to eliminate some food allergies. This brought further improvement.

My work with Julie demonstrates how a comprehensive approach to Lyme disease can help to overcome this illness. The Chinese herbs I recommend helped reduce her Lyme load by killing the organism. They also helped improve her circulation while supporting her immune system.

As I've mentioned in previous chapters, antibiotics can suppress the body's own immunity. Fortunately, the herbs in the protocols in this chapter have the opposite effect. They actually support your immune system in fighting the infection. Since doctors currently lack a technology that measures your body's actual Lyme load, the reduction of Lyme signs and symptoms is the best marker of success. As you become symptom-free, you clear a major hurdle in Lyme disease. The aim of all the recommendations in this chapter is to get you there.

The Five Protocols for Treating Lyme

It's long been drummed into us that all people who have one specific disease will be cured by the very same pill. As a result, people (and even many conventional doctors) overlook the reality that each one of us is biochemically unique. That's why even if it works for other folks, there is no way of exactly predicting whether a treatment will work for you. In my practice, most of my patients get favorable results from the first treatment option I will offer you in this chapter. But some people do better on other protocols. So I will offer you all five protocols that I've seen work for people with Lyme disease. After this introduction to the protocols, I'll let you know how to proceed to use them to find out which Lyme solution is right for you.

The Zhang Protocol

I was introduced to Dr. Qingcai Zhang in New York City in 2003, after my many failed courses of antibiotics. I had heard about him from other people he treated successfully for Lyme disease. Dr. Zhang has more than fifty years' experience treating chronic infections, including Lyme, HIV, and hepatitis C. He extensively researched spirochete diseases in China in order to develop herbal formulas that can help alleviate Lyme disease symptoms and regulate immune function. Dr. Zhang has coined the term *modern Chinese medicine*, which combines the tenets of traditional Chinese medicine with his knowledge of the biological activity of Chinese herbs.

Chinese herbal formulas are designed to work in harmony with each other in order to minimize side effects while delivering the desired clinical outcome. These herbal combinations have broader effects than just using herbs singly. Dr. Zhang's formulas specifically address the multitude of symptoms Lyme disease creates.

I have personally used his formulas and treated thousands of people with them, too. In my experience, they have often provided relief when other treatments have failed. The formulas are generally very well tolerated and side effects are rare. These are my "go-to" herbs with adults and teens that have Lyme disease. I have seen many people recover using these herbs. While they are highly effective, they are also somewhat expensive, so they may be cost-prohibitive for some people. It is a good investment in your health, but if the herbs are not affordable for you, please use the Modified Cowden Protocol.

The Cowden Protocol

Dr. Lee Cowden is a retired cardiologist in Dallas, Texas, who years ago developed this herbal protocol after successfully treating a young man with chronic Lyme disease. The patient had not responded to antibiotics but had significant improvement after taking the herbs that Dr. Cowden recommended. After that, Dr. Cowden began to use these herbs successfully with other people. He developed several liquid herbal formulas that contain special local herbs from Peru or nearby areas of South America. Local healers used these plants for many generations and knew a great deal about each herb's healing properties. Despite these herbs' long-standing traditional use, only recently have Western doctors begun to understand their unique biochemical properties.

Known as the Cowden Protocol, this treatment takes five to nine months. During that time, you will take combinations of thirteen different herbal formulas. Each month, the protocol changes slightly. A comprehensive program that also effectively kills Lyme disease and co-infections, this protocol has special features that are most helpful for people who have not responded well to (or could not tolerate) the Zhang Protocol, including people who may be allergic to some of the ingredients, and children, who cannot swallow capsules easily. I have actually used a modified version of the Cowden protocol that I will discuss in more detail below.

Byron White Formulas

Byron White, a natural health practitioner, developed several formulas to treat Lyme disease, tick-borne co-infections, Candida, Epstein-Barr virus, and many other infectious agents. His formulas are very potent.

Even a few drops can have strong effects. Some practitioners like these herbs because you only need to use a few drops one to two times a day, which is easy to manage for most Lyme patients. However, some people experience a reaction to the rapid detox in these formulas, so it's not a first-choice protocol on my plan.

Stephen Buhner Protocol

The herbalist Stephen Buhner developed an effective protocol that uses Japanese knotwood (*Polygonum cuspidatum*), cat's claw (*Uncaria tomentosa*), and andrographis (*Andrographis paniculata*) to eliminate Lyme disease and the co-infections. Many other herbs are part of his extended protocol. I have more clinical success with Dr. Zhang's or Dr. Cowden's protocol, but if other treatments have not been tolerated or successful, this is always an option. Don't get discouraged if your symptoms do not improve as quickly as you'd like! Be persistent in finding the best path to recovery.

Beyond Balance Protocol

These herbal products were developed by Susan McCamish. Although there is no specific protocol, these herbal formulas can be combined to help eradicate Lyme and coinfections. Most of the products are liquid extracts, although some are capsules. As with the Byron White formulas, these are potent, even in drop doses, and can definitely cause detox reactions (discussed later in this chapter). They are currently sold only to health-care providers, so you would need to work with someone who uses these products to start this protocol.

Protocols for Treating Active Lyme Disease

Each of the protocols that follow is designed to ease the burden of Lyme and other bacterial load on your body. They will simultaneously reduce inflammation, improve circulation, stop the formation of abnormal immune reactions in the body, and help modulate a healthy immune response to the microbe. Although there are many different treatments to help individuals with Lyme disease, I am offering you the ones with which I've had the greatest clinical success in working with thousands of people. I will also emphasize the ones that have the least side effects.

The recommendations for both acute and chronic Lyme differ slightly, as you will see. Depending on whether you were recently diagnosed with Lyme disease or have had it for many years, follow the instructions for either acute or chronic to get yourself back on the right track.

I always recommend that people (except for children under age eight) begin with the Zhang Protocol because it's the most successful in helping my patients with Lyme disease recover. It was also the protocol that helped me overcome my Lyme disease.

Later in this chapter, I will explain the known properties and benefits of each herb used in the different protocols. This will help you understand exactly how the recommended herbal protocols resolve Lyme by boosting the immune system and reducing your Lyme load. These are powerhouse herbs and, when taken in the combinations recommended, they are game-changers in recovering from Lyme disease.

The basic instructions will show you exactly how to proceed with each protocol:

- How to begin
- Which protocol to try first

- Which supplements to take
- How long to take the protocol
- How to evaluate whether you need to continue on the protocol
- How to determine when you would benefit by changing to another protocol—along with guidance for which protocol to use next

Most people want to know which protocol will work best for them. Unfortunately, there is no way to predict that without trying the protocols first. This is why I offer a sequence and parameters that help you figure out your most effective treatment.

Quick Guide to Treatment Protocols

The acute and chronic protocols differ, so which one should you follow? Here are some basic guidelines.

You should follow the Acute Lyme Disease Protocol if:

- You have recently been diagnosed with Lyme by a health-care professional.
- You have recently been diagnosed with Lyme using the Lyme Disease Symptom Questionnaire (page 42).
- You are experiencing the acute-phase symptoms detailed in Chapter 1 on page 12.
- You have recently been bitten by a tick (or other insect bite associated with transmitting Lyme).
- You have noted a bull's-eye rash.
- You decide to undertake an herbal protocol rather than undergo the initial twenty-one-day antibiotic treatment, or

you wish to take herbs in addition to the twenty-one days of antibiotics.

You should follow the Chronic Lyme Disease Protocol if:

- You are experiencing the chronic-phase symptoms detailed in Chapter 1 on page 13.
- You have been experiencing Lyme symptoms for three months or more.

Acute Lyme Disease Protocol

How to Begin

For adults and children over age eight, I recommend that you start with the Zhang Protocol unless you cannot swallow capsules or have a known allergy to one of the components in the formulas. Please check the ingredients to find out. The products can be obtained from my store at dariningelsnd.com/store. If you cannot swallow capsules or are allergic to any of the Zhang ingredients, please take the Modified Cowden Protocol as directed. Children under age eight should always use the Modified Cowden Protocol. Because of differences in metabolism and weight, the correct dosage will depend on your age—just as occurs with drug prescriptions. In the following sections you will find more information about each component of the protocol.

With all protocols, I recommend that you simultaneously do the biofilm protocol detailed in this chapter on page 151. (I explain why the biofilm protocol enhances the effectiveness of the main protocol on page 158.)

In my instructions, you will notice that I mention Herxheimer reactions (detox reactions), which some people experience. They may or may not happen, but it's important to be able to recognize them if they occur.

The Jarisch-Herxheimer Reaction

The Jarisch-Herxheimer reaction, better known as a Herx reaction or *herxing*, is the body's response to a die-off of bacteria, such as Lyme spirochetes, that occurs more quickly than the body can remove them. The reaction feels flu-like, with more fatigue, joint pain, headaches, muscle aches, anxiety, heart palpitations, fever, chills, flushing, and rapid heart rate. It can be extremely uncomfortable and, if you are not prepared for it, very worrisome. When you experience herxing, it's natural to feel that something else is wrong with you. As uncomfortable as it may be, a Herx reaction usually indicates that the treatment is working.

Based on years of guiding my patients, I recommend continuing with the treatment despite the herxing. To make the herxing symptoms more manageable, you can decrease the dose of your herbs for three weeks and see if your symptoms improve. If the herxing is becoming unbearable, you can take two capsules of AI#3 three times a day (if on the Zhang Protocol) or ten drops of Burbur every two hours until your symptoms get better (if on the Cowden Protocol). Once the herxing stops, many people feel significantly better. Herx reactions can last from a few days to a few weeks. On page 150 of this chapter you will find a more comprehensive protocol for treating a Herx reaction.

Plan on being on the Zhang Protocol (or, alternatively, the Modified Cowden Protocol) for at least six weeks. Once you start treatment, you should begin to feel better fairly quickly, but it is important to take the herbs for at least six weeks to ensure that you have killed the infection, even if you feel better sooner.

If you still have symptoms at the end of six weeks but are experiencing improvement, then continue on the regimen for another four to six weeks, for a total of about three months.

If there has been no change in your symptoms after six weeks, then you may need to use a different protocol. If you started with the Zhang Protocol, please start the Modified Cowden Protocol. If you started with the Modified Cowden Protocol, then I would recommend using the Zhang Protocol. If you have tried both the Zhang Protocol and the Modified Cowden Protocol, then I would try one of the other herbal protocols listed in this chapter.

Recommendations for Adults (Under Age Sixty-Five)

Take Dr. Zhang's HH Caps, Coptis, and Cordyceps. Take one capsule three times a day. You may add allicin if you tolerate garlic and do not find the odor offensive. Add AI#3 (one capsule three times per day) if you experience joint or muscle pain. Add Puerarin Caps (one capsule three times per day) if you have high fever, muscle aches, or Raynaud's syndrome.

If you cannot swallow capsules, please use the Modified Cowden Protocol. Take Samento, Banderol, and Cumanda, thirty drops two times a day in 1 ounce of water. You may add ten drops of Burbur every thirty minutes if you start to get Herx reactions.

Recommendations for Adults (Age Sixty-Five and Older)

Take Dr. Zhang's HH Caps, Coptis, and Cordyceps, one capsule two times a day. Add AI#3 (one capsule two times per day) if you experience joint or muscle pain. Add Puerarin Caps (one capsule two times per day) if you have high fever, muscle aches, or Raynaud's syndrome. These same herbs are used for adults under age sixty-five. I use a lower dose since many people in this age group have other underlying health problems, such as kidney or liver disease. Or they may be taking medications that would alter how the herbs get metabolized.

If you cannot swallow capsules, please use the Modified Cowden Protocol. Take Samento, Banderol, and Cumanda, fifteen drops two times a day in 1 ounce of water. You may add five drops of Burbur every thirty minutes if you start to get Herx reactions. If you have poor kidney or liver function, then please discuss dosing with your doctor before starting any herbal regimen.

Recommendations for Teens and Children (Age Eight and Older)

If your child can swallow capsules, he or she can take Dr. Zhang's HH Caps, Coptis, and Cordyceps, one capsule two times a day. Add AI#3 (one capsule two times per day) if your child experiences joint or muscle pain. Add Puerarin Caps (one capsule two times per day) if your child has high fever, muscle aches, or Raynaud's syndrome.

If your child is unable to swallow capsules, please use the Modified Cowden Protocol. He or she can take Samento, Banderol, and Cumanda, fifteen drops two times a day in 1 ounce of water. You may add five drops of Burbur every thirty minutes if your child starts to get Herx reactions.

Recommendations for Children (Under Age Eight)

Use the Modified Cowden Protocol. Have your child take Samento, Banderol, and Cumanda, five to six drops two times a day in 1 ounce of water. You may add two to three drops of Burbur every thirty minutes if your child starts to get Herx reactions.

Chronic Lyme Disease Protocol

How to Begin

Start with the Zhang Protocol as listed, or you can use the Modified Cowden Protocol if you cannot swallow capsules or are allergic to one of the components in the formulas. If you experience Herx reactions, follow the guidelines on managing the symptoms to get you through it a little easier.

How Long to Continue

Plan on being on this treatment protocol for at least three months. The progress tends to be slow for most people, and there will be ups and downs in your symptoms during this time.

　　If you see improvement at the end of three months but are still having symptoms, then continue with the protocol for another three months. You can safely stay on this protocol for as long as a year, with the exception of the Dr. Zhang product AI#3. This product should be temporarily discontinued (for reasons discussed later in this chapter). It's best to feel well for at least one month before you stop taking the herbs.

When to Change Protocols

If you started with the Zhang Protocol and have not noticed any improvement after three months, then start the Modified Cowden Protocol. I have had some patients that seem to do better with one protocol over another for no apparent reason, so it's worth trying a different treatment if one protocol is not giving you relief from your symptoms. If you have taken the Zhang Protocol herbs and the Modified Cowden Protocol herbs and still do not feel well, then it's time to move to the Byron White herbs or the Beyond Balance products. Don't get discouraged! I find that most of my patients respond well to one of the herbal protocols, so you just need to find what works best for you.

Recommendations for Adults (Under Age Sixty-Five)

Take Dr. Zhang's HH Caps, Artemisiae Caps, Circulation P, Cordyceps, and R-5081. Take one capsule three times a day. Add AI#3 (one capsule three times per day) if you experience joint or muscle pain. Add Puerarin Caps (one capsule three times per day) if you have high fever, muscle aches, or Raynaud's syndrome.

If you cannot swallow capsules, use the Modified Cowden Protocol. Take Samento, Banderol, and Cumanda, starting with two drops two times a day in 1 ounce of water. If you do not feel any improvement, you may increase by one drop two times a day, every three days, up to thirty drops two times a day. If you start to feel better, then do not increase the dose. If you start to get a Herx reaction, do not increase or decrease your dose, but keep it exactly as is. You can add ten drops of Burbur every thirty minutes if you start to get Herx reactions.

Recommendations for Adults
(Age Sixty-Five or Older)

Take Dr. Zhang's HH Caps, Artemisiae Caps, Coptis, Cordyceps, and R-5081. Take one capsule two times a day. Add AI#3 (one capsule two times per day) if you experience joint or muscle pain. Add Puerarin Caps (one capsule two times per day) if you have high fever, muscle aches, or Raynaud's syndrome.

If you cannot swallow capsules, then use the Modified Cowden Protocol. Take Samento, Banderol, and Cumanda, starting with one drop two times a day in 1 ounce of water. If you do not feel any improvement, you may increase by one drop two times a day, every three days, up to fifteen drops two times a day. If you start to feel better, then do not increase the dose. If you start to get a Herx reaction, do not increase or decrease your dose, but keep it where it is. You can add five drops of Burbur every thirty minutes if you start to get Herx reactions. If you have poor kidney or liver function, then please discuss dosing with your doctor before starting any herbal regimen.

Recommendations for Teens and Children
(Age Eight and Older)

If your child can swallow capsules, he or she can take Dr. Zhang's HH Caps, Artemisiae Caps, Circulation P, Cordyceps, and R-5081, one capsule two times a day. Add AI#3 (one capsule two times per day) if your child experiences joint or muscle pain. Add Puerarin Caps (one capsule two times per day) if your child has high fever, muscle aches, or Raynaud's syndrome.

If your child cannot swallow capsules, please use the Modified Cowden Protocol. Have your child take Samento, Banderol, and

Cumanda, starting with one drop two times a day in 1 ounce of water. If your child does not feel any improvement, you may increase by one drop two times a day, every three days, up to fifteen drops two times a day. If your child starts to feel better, then do not increase the dose. If he or she starts to get a Herx reaction, do not increase or decrease the dose, but keep it where it is. You can add five drops of Burbur every thirty minutes if your child starts to get Herx reactions.

Recommendations for Children (Under Age Eight)

Use the Modified Cowden Protocol. He or she can take Samento, Banderol, and Cumanda, starting with one drop two times a day in 1 ounce of water. If your child does not feel any improvement, you may increase by one drop two times a day, every three days, up to ten drops two times a day. If your child starts to feel better, then do not increase the dose. If he or she starts to get a Herx reaction, do not increase or decrease the dose, but keep it where it is. You can add five drops of Burbur every thirty minutes if your child starts to get Herx reactions.

Dr. Zhang's Supplements

Chinese herbal medicine differs significantly from Western herbal medicine. Chinese herbology typically combines herbs into formulas containing a dozen or more different herbs, whereas Western herbs are often used individually to treat a specific symptom or condition. In order to understand how these supplements can help, please familiarize yourself with the properties of Dr. Zhang's formulas.

ALLICIN CAPSULES

Garlic has a long history as an antimicrobial. Called *Russian penicillin,* it was carried by Russian soldiers during World War I to treat illness or wounds sustained in the field. Garlic's many health benefits include reducing cholesterol, improving circulation, enhancing detoxification, and reducing inflammation. Its success at treating bacterial, yeast, and some parasite infections is well documented.[1] The many types of readily available garlic supplements do not all produce the same results. For example, "odorless" garlic extracts, available from several companies, do not effectively kill microbes.[2]

Allicin, an active ingredient in garlic, which is responsible for its strong odor, is highly effective at reducing the bacterial load for both Lyme disease and its co-infections such as *Babesia.*[3] Allicin capsules are a concentrated extract of allitridi, which the body converts to allicin.

Allicin capsules are time-released, so the product disperses evenly throughout the gut. Because it will be absorbed over a longer period of time, blood levels of allicin will stay elevated longer, giving them a better chance to kill the Lyme organism.

Research has shown that allicin and allitridi are extremely safe, with no known toxicity.[4] However, allicin capsules are not appropriate for anyone who is allergic to garlic or has difficulty with sulfur-containing foods, such as eggs, legumes, and cruciferous vegetables like broccoli, cauliflower, and cabbage. If you are sensitive to sulfur-containing foods, they will usually give you gas, bloating, abdominal pain, and bowel changes after you eat them. If you experience these reactions, you can omit taking allicin.

When taking allicin, most people notice a change in their body odor, since the allicin is broken down and ultimately excreted in the skin. For some, this can be difficult to tolerate and socially challenging. To try to reduce it, you can take 100 milligrams of chlorophyll with the allicin capsules.

ARTEMISIAE CAPSULES

Primarily an extract of wormwood, Artemisiae (*Artemisia annua*) capsules are widely used because of their efficacy in treating malaria.[5] Babesiosis (*Babesia species*), a common co-infection with Lyme disease, is caused by a blood parasite closely related to malaria. Artemisiae capsules also contain extracts of astragalus (*Astragalus membranaceus*) and codonopsis (*Codonopsis pilosula*). This herbal combination helps fight off infection while regulating the immune system. In animal studies, Artemisiae capsules have been shown to suppress the production of autoantibodies and reduce inflammatory molecules.[6] This may help to block some of the autoimmune reactivity that occurs with Lyme disease, as well as killing off some of the microbes.

Most people tolerate Artemisiae capsules even when used for extended lengths of time. The astragalus in the formula helps reduce inflammation, regulates the immune system, and generates potent antioxidant activity. Codonopsis is primarily an adaptogenic herb, which means it helps your body defend itself against high levels of stress, anxiety, or fatigue. It is also helpful if you are experiencing flare-ups of autoimmune symptoms, especially joint pain, skin rashes, and neuropathy.

AI#3 CAPSULES

This highly effective combination of *Macunae caulis*, *Sargentodoxae caulis*, and *Paederiae caulis* is one of the best anti-inflammatories available. In addition, it is an effective analgesic, so it helps reduce pain. It can be used with other inflammatory conditions, such as rheumatoid arthritis, Crohn's disease, and psoriasis. AI#3 helps reduce inflammation rather quickly without the risk of stomach ulcers or gastrointestinal distress that can occur with other nonsteroidal anti-inflammatory drugs (NSAIDs), such as ibuprofen or naproxen sodium. Use it if your symptoms include joint or muscle pain, fibromyalgia, or headache, or if you are experiencing severe Herx reactions. Although other herbs are more effective at helping people fall or stay asleep, AI#3 also has mild sedating effects, so it can help if your sleep is disturbed.

Because of the immune-suppressive nature of AI#3, it's best not to take it for more than three to four months at a time. Although this formula is nontoxic, it can sometimes cause irregularities of the menstrual cycle, so women should stop using it at least three months prior to trying to conceive.

Take the capsules as listed earlier for pain and inflammation. If the inflammation gets significantly worse, increase the dose to two capsules in the morning, one capsule in the afternoon, and two capsules in the evening for at least three to five days until the symptoms improve. Then resume the standard dose.

CIRCULATION P CAPSULES

This ten-herb combination is a modified version of two traditional Chinese herbal formulas that help improve circulation. Historically, these formulas were used to help with cold hands and feet, dark circles around the eyes, moles, dry skin or rashes, and abdominal pain. Since blood flow is often restricted in people with Lyme disease, this formula helps open up the small blood vessels, allowing for more nutrients, oxygen, and immune cells to get to the right areas of the body.

Circulation P can prevent platelet stickiness, the first step in clot formation. When platelets stick together, the blood becomes thicker, making it more difficult to pass through the smaller blood vessels. However, unlike a true blood thinner like warfarin or heparin, Circulation P does not impair your ability to clot if you get cut or injured. In addition to improving blood flow, this formula also enhances immune function by helping your tissues' immune cells more readily rid the body of bacteria and viruses.[7]

This formula is often effective for those with chronic cold hands and feet, numbness and tingling, brain fog, poor memory, or chronic intestinal problems. It also seems to work well for persistent inflammation, especially joint pain. It can reduce the swelling and heal the inflamed tissue. After surgery, it can promote faster healing, since better circulation brings more nutrients to the damaged areas of the body.

COPTIS CAPSULES

Coptis (*Coptis chinensis*) is used to treat various infections, including bacteria, viruses, yeast, and parasites. Studies have found it as effective as some common antibiotics in stopping the growth of harmful bacteria.[8] It has historically been used to treat intestinal infections, stomach infections, and deep skin infections. Coptis has also been used for upper respiratory infections, such as bronchitis or sinusitis.

Because of its broad antimicrobial effects, as you learned in Chapter 2, I also recommend taking coptis as soon as you realize a Lyme tick has bitten you. This is helpful when it's too early to do a blood test. Coptis can potentially help eradicate any of the tick-borne microbes before they start to trigger symptoms.

Many people with Lyme disease also have other viral infections, such as Epstein-Barr virus or human herpes-6 virus (HHV-6). Persistent viruses can cause fatigue, pain, numbness, or tingling or swollen glands. Many of these viruses are opportunistic, which means that they become active when your immune system is suppressed. Keeping them in check is important for maintaining better health. Coptis is an excellent way to help reduce viral load, so these viruses are less likely to produce troublesome symptoms.

CORDYCEPS CAPSULES

Cordyceps (*Cordyceps sinensis*) has been used in Chinese medicine for over two thousand years. A type of mushroom that is found only in a very small part of China, it has many benefits, including improving blood flow, increasing white blood cell count, and enhancing immune activity.[9] Cordyceps is good for people with Lyme who are completely run down and need a little more pep in their step. If you are dealing with chronic fatigue syndrome and fibromyalgia, where persistent fatigue is common, it can be quite useful.

There has been quite a bit of research on cordyceps, especially with regard to chronic hepatitis, HIV, tuberculosis, and other viral infections. Cordyceps's immune-boosting effects make it ideal to address immune deficiency or improve immune function. Because of its effects on blood flow, cordyceps can also help reduce high blood pressure.[10]

HH CAPSULES

The main herb in this formula is *Houttuynia cordata*, a well-established Chinese herb used to treat various types of bacterial and fungal infections. In addition to its antimicrobial effects, *Houttuynia* helps boost immune function and reduce swelling and is anti-inflammatory. It is metabolized rapidly in the body, so it's important to take it three times per day to maintain blood levels.

Because of its antimicrobial benefits, I use this formula for both acute and chronic Lyme disease as well as other coinfections. There is no known toxicity and is safe for both children and adults.

R-5081 CAPSULES

A traditional Chinese seven-herb formula, R-5081 features *Scutellariae radix* and *Smilax glabra*, used for years to treat syphilis and leptospira, both of which are spirochete infections, like Lyme. The other herbs in the formula supply additional antimicrobial activity, reduce inflammation, enhance detoxification, and help promote tissue repair.[11]

Use this formula to help support the immune system and eradicate underlying infection. There is no known toxicity to any of the herbs, so this formula can be used long-term.

PUERARIN CAPSULES

The root of the *Pueraria species* has traditionally been used to treat high fever, muscle spasms, headaches, stiff joints, and diarrhea. Because it has been shown to help improve blood flow to the heart and brain, it is particularly good for those experiencing brain fog or poor memory.[12] Pueraria also help reduce blood pressure and serve as a mild blood thinner. People who have persistent migraines, headaches, or chest pain can especially benefit from Puerarin. Note: If you experience chest pain, see a cardiologist for evaluation, to make sure it is nothing serious or life-threatening. Do not take any herbal product until your health-care provider has determined it is safe for you.

People with Raynaud's syndrome can also benefit from these capsules. In Reynaud's, which is common in people with Lyme, particularly women, the hands and feet are cold and blue in appearance because of lack of blood. This condition is often mistaken for other heart or blood vessel problems.

ANGEL'S STORY

Angel was a stellar high school student athlete. Several colleges scouted her to play softball. Unfortunately, in her senior year, she began to experience fatigue and joint pain in her knees. It got so bad, she had trouble walking some days. To rule out rheumatoid arthritis and lupus, her primary-care doctor ran some basic blood tests, which came back negative. Then, over the next several months, the joint pain began affecting her hips, ankles, and shoulders. She missed several softball games because of pain. Without identifying any underlying cause, the rheumatologist she consulted prescribed powerful steroids to calm the inflammation.

They provided only mild relief. Angel started looking for other answers.

When Angel came to our clinic, she was visibly in pain and had difficulty walking. Her knees were swollen and red. Her skin was flushed all over. She said that she had looked this way for months, that she was having difficulty getting her school-work done, and that her memory was not as sharp as it had been in the past. She was always tired and really never had "good days." I reviewed all of her previous labs, which were mostly normal. I asked if she had ever been tested for Lyme disease. It turned out that out of all the doctors she had seen, no one had looked into it. Again, here was an individual who lived in Massachusetts and had spent time outdoors in a region known to carry deer ticks. After I ran several tests for Lyme disease and co-infections, her labs came back positive for Lyme and babesiosis.

I started Angel on Artemisiae, HH Capsules, AI#3, Circulation P, Coptis, and R-5081. She also began a biofilm protocol (see later in this chapter) and took the recommended nutrients to help support her immune system. After a week on the Chinese herbs and nutrients, her joint pain started to subside, her knees looked less swollen, her energy had improved, and it was easier for her to get through the school day. We continued on this regimen for three months. Each week she continued to improve. She had some Herx reactions periodically over the course of treatment, but these passed after a few days.

By the fourth month, Angel's symptoms were 90 percent better. I made a small change in her protocol. I added Cordyceps capsules to help with her energy, which markedly improved in the next few weeks. Angel is now in college and has been feeling well. She has had one flare-up since going away to school but was able to manage with a short course of Chinese herbs, and she is now an active, happy college student.

The Cowden Protocol

If you have started on the Zhang Protocol with no improvement after three months of treatment (or you have difficulty tolerating the herbal supplements), then the next step is to use my Modified Cowden Protocol.

It helps break down biofilm (see later in this chapter), reduces inflammation, improves detoxification, and helps modulate immune function. Like the Zhang Protocol, it addresses many of the chronic problems that Lyme disease creates and has helped many people with whom I've worked.

Many of my patients with Lyme disease like the Cowden Protocol, because it is primarily made up of liquid extracts that are easy to administer. Each herbal formula is given in drop doses, so they can be carefully prescribed to meet each individual's target dose.

These highly concentrated herbs are potent even when using a few drops at a time. Because they are so strong, I often start with very small amounts and increase the dose as tolerated. Some people get Herx reactions with only one or two drops of a specific formula. With Lyme, sometimes less is more. It is always easy to start small and increase doses as you feel you can tolerate more.

For many people with Lyme disease, the full Cowden Protocol can be cumbersome and difficult to follow. The protocol changes every month, so people must keep track of the different herbs, which also must be taken at specific times of day. This is designed to treat Lyme in its different forms and to aid in detoxification. If you have brain fog, as many people with Lyme do, that can be challenging. The easier the treatment, the better. Having worked with the Cowden Protocol over the years, I have developed my own modified version of it, which primarily uses four herbal formulas. I have found this to be both effective and simpler for most people with Lyme to manage. It consists of the following four herbs.

SAMENTO

Samento is an extract of cat's claw (*Uncaria tomentosa*), which is one of the most effective herbs against Lyme disease, even when used by itself. The extract comes from a woody vine that grows primarily in the Amazon rain forests. Indigenous people have used cat's claw for more than two thousand years. It also helps eradicate many other tick-borne infections such as *Babesia, Bartonella, Ehrlichia, Mycoplasma*, and *Rickettsia*. A potent anti-inflammatory, cat's claw can help reduce joint pain, headaches, muscle aches, abdominal pain, and inflammatory skin rashes associated with Lyme disease. I have often prescribed Samento for other inflammatory conditions including Crohn's disease, ulcerative colitis, arthritis, sciatica, and asthma. Samento is effective at reducing inflammation with little to no side effects.

While there are several cat's claw extracts on the market, Samento is especially rich in compounds called pentacyclic oxindole alkaloids (POAs). These stimulate the immune system to fight off the infection. Many cat's claw extracts contain a mixture of POAs and tetracyclic oxindole alkaloids (TOAs). There is some controversy about whether using a TOA-free extract is superior to using one that contains both POAs and TOAs. Evidence suggests that the TOAs may inhibit the immune-stimulating benefits of POAs. Samento is TOA-free, so the active POAs have the best chance to activate the immune system. Samento often works where other cat's claw extracts have failed.

Because Samento is a powerful formula, Herx reactions are common, even when starting with small doses. Start with three to four drops twice a day in 1 ounce of water, and then increase the dose every three to four days by one drop twice a day. You can incrementally increase to up to thirty drops twice a day if needed. Most people start to feel a difference when they take ten to fifteen drops twice a day. If you start to experience a Herx reaction, don't increase the dose. There is no benefit to increasing the dose, as the reaction will likely only worsen. For children, start with one drop twice a day in 1 ounce of water and increase as tolerated.

BANDEROL

Banderol comes from another native tree (*Otaba species*) found in the rain forests of Peru and other parts of South America. Like Samento, it has broad-spectrum activity against bacteria, viruses, yeast, and parasites. It helps kill Lyme disease and co-infections, so it works well in conjunction with Samento to reduce the load of organisms in your body. Banderol has some anti-inflammatory benefits as well.

Eva Sapi, PhD, and her group of researchers at the University of New Haven found that the combination of Samento and Banderol was effective at killing all three forms of *Borrelia burgdorferi* (the Lyme bacteria) in test-tube studies.[13] The three forms of the bacteria are the spirochete, cyst, and cell-wall deficient—meaning it has no cell walls, making it difficult for antibiotics to attack. The researchers also discovered that doxycycline, the most commonly prescribed antibiotic for Lyme disease, was effective at killing *Borrelia burgdorferi* only when it was in its full spirochete form. Although this was only a test-tube study, it suggests that unlike doxycycline, these herbs are able to treat Lyme in its many different stages. As with Samento, start with three to four drops twice a day in 1 ounce of water and then increase the dose every three to four days by 1 drop twice a day, up to thirty drops twice a day if needed. Herx reactions can also occur with Banderol, although less than with Samento. For children, start with one drop twice a day in 1 ounce of water and increase as tolerated.

CUMANDA

Continuing with the quartet of antimicrobial herbs in my Modified Cowden Protocol is Cumanda (*Campsiandra angustifolia*), which comes from the bark of an Amazonian tree. This herb may have the broadest activity against microbes of all the formulas in the protocol. Cumanda has been used to treat many infections, including Lyme disease, hepatitis, Candida, and parasites, and has been used by native populations as a treatment for malaria. A strong anti-inflammatory, it has also traditionally been used for arthritis and reducing fever.

Out of the three herbs in the Modified Cowden Protocol, this one seems to be most likely to trigger Herx reactions. Start with three to four drops twice a day in 1 ounce of water and then increase the dose by one drop twice a day, up to thirty drops twice a day if needed. I find that I usually need to increase the dose much more slowly than with Samento or Banderol. Instead of increasing it every three to four days, try increasing the dose every seven to ten days. This way, there is less likelihood of having a Herx reaction, and you will still get the herb's antimicrobial and anti-inflammatory benefits. For children, start with one drop twice a day in 1 ounce of water and increase as tolerated.

BURBUR

· ·

Burbur is made from the leaves of *Desmodium molliculum*, a native South American plant. Where the combination of Samento, Banderol, and Cumanda is designed to eradicate Lyme disease, reduce inflammation, and modulate the immune system, Burbur has a different purpose as part of the protocol. This herbal preparation helps aid the body in detoxifying. It specifically helps detoxify the kidneys, liver, and lymphatic system. Burbur can help protect the liver against outside toxins, such as some pharmaceuticals, chemicals, and mold toxins.

I recommend that you also use Burbur in conjunction with the other three herbs on the Modified Cowden Protocol. Burbur greatly diminishes the die-off effects from the antimicrobial herbs. If the Herx reactions are severe, you can take Burbur more frequently until the symptoms lessen or go away completely. Start with ten drops twice a day in 1 ounce of water. You can increase up to ten drops every thirty minutes if necessary to control the Herx reactions. Since you don't want to stop the antimicrobial herbs if you're experiencing a Herx reaction, Burbur makes the treatment more tolerable.

Other Herbal Therapies

Many other herbal therapies have worked well for people with Lyme disease. If you have started an herbal protocol and given it six months, and still don't feel better, then move on to a different herbal protocol.

If the plan you first selected is working, within three months of starting the treatment, you will begin noticing less joint pain or muscle aches, better energy, less brain fog, fewer headaches, and an improved overall sense of well-being. Even if these signs of improvement are small, they indicate that you are on the right track and should continue with the regimen. Often you will start to feel much better in sooner than three months. However, if your symptoms are no better or even worse than when you started your herbs, it is a good idea to try a different protocol. Sometimes one protocol works better than another for no logical reason, so it's worth trying another herbal regimen if you're not getting the results you and your doctor want.

Given the complexity of Lyme disease, many organisms, forms, and immune factors affect the results a person will get from each therapy. You will be the best judge of what's right for you—and if you are unsure, consult a physician in the book's Resources section (page 325).

Byron White Formulas

As mentioned earlier, the Byron White formulas are quite potent. As a result, herxing is quite common with these formulas. The virtue of these formulas is that it's possible to target specific Lyme-related infections. Since each formula is specific to the infection you are trying to treat, knowing what infection(s) you have is important. Consult with a physician about testing to ensure that you take the correct herbs that correspond to the specific infections. For example:

- A-L complex is used to treat Lyme disease.
- A-Bab is used to treat *Babesia*.
- A-Bart is used to treat *Bartonella*.
- A-Bio is used to treat *Ehrlichia* and other bacterial infections.
- A-EB/H6 is used to treat herpes viruses, such as Epstein-Barr (mono), herpes simplex, cytomegalovirus, and varicella-zoster (chicken pox/shingles).
- A-Myco is used to treat *Mycoplasma*.

- A-P is used to treat parasites.
- A-RMSF is used to treat Rocky Mountain Spotted Fever.
- A-FNG is used to treat Candida and other fungal infections.
- A-V is used to treat other viruses.

Start with only one drop a day in 1 ounce of water. You can increase the dose every three days by one drop, if tolerated, up to fifteen drops a day. Some of my patients have tolerated and needed higher amounts, but most people respond at lower doses. If either you start to herx or you start to feel better, maintain the same dose. You should increase the dose only if there is no response at all.

How to Prevent and Reduce Herxing

You can take any one of the following anti-inflammatory or detoxifying herbs to prevent, reduce, or minimize Herx reactions, no matter which protocol you are following. Follow these recommendations until the reactions subside, which is usually within a few days. If the herxing lasts longer, you can take them until you feel comfortable again.

- AI#3: One capsule three to four times per day before meals.
- Burbur: Ten drops every fifteen to thirty minutes in 1 ounce of water.
- Curcumin (*Curcuma longa*): This is derived from turmeric. Curcumin can be difficult to absorb, so not all products are created equal. I recommend only products that have been manufactured to increase absorption, such as Meriva from Thorne Research, Theracurmin HP from Integrated Therapeutics, or my own specially formulated curcumin extract,

available in my online store. Take two to three capsules two
to three times per day before meals.

- Boswellia (*Boswellia serrata*), 400 milligrams: This is an herb
  from India with a long history of use as an anti-inflammatory.
  Take one to two capsules three times per day before meals.
- White willow bark (*Salix alba*), 400 milligrams: This herb
  contains salicin, a component similar to that found in aspirin.
  Take one to two capsules three times per day before meals.

Alkalinizing your body will also help keep herxing under control.
You can take a bicarbonate formula to help keep you more alkaline. I
recommend taking either:

- Alka Seltzer Gold: One tablet three to four times per day in
  2 to 4 ounces of water.
- Tri-Salts: Two capsules three times per day.

If your Herx reactions become unbearable, discuss this with your
health-care provider so he or she can alter your treatment plan to keep
you moving forward.

Busting the Biofilm: How to Eliminate the Slime

Do you ever wake up with thick, white, slimy gunk on your teeth? This
gunk has a name: biofilm. Produced by bacteria, it consists of a matrix
of carbohydrates, proteins, and other cellular products. Although scientists still lack complete knowledge as to how or why biofilm forms,
there are a few working theories. One scenario is that bacteria adhere

to cell surfaces to provide the organism with a protective layer against its own immune system. This prevents the immune system from attacking bacteria that *belong* in the body. However, biofilm production may also play a role in antibiotic resistance. Urinary tract infections, ear infections, heart valve problems, gingivitis, and many hospital-acquired infections are related to biofilm.

In the treatment of Lyme disease, the thick biofilm layer shields the bacteria from the immune system, thereby preventing antibodies as well as herbs and antibiotics from penetrating the cell wall. Research suggests that killing biofilm-coated bacteria would require a higher-magnitude dose (100 to 1,000 times higher) than would be needed to kill one *without* the biofilm covering.[14] Lyme disease produces loads of biofilm, one reason it's such a difficult infection to treat. To make things worse, there is some evidence that antibiotics may actually increase Lyme's biofilm production.[15] On the other hand, if you can break down the biofilm naturally, the protocols can work more effectively to kill the Lyme infection. That's why destroying the slime is essential to Lyme disease treatment.

Anju Usman, MD, of Naperville, Illinois, is one of the foremost experts on biofilm, and I primarily use her protocol. To strip away the slime, take the supplements listed here at least an hour before consuming or using any mineral-containing products that may interfere with stripping the biofilm. Avoid multivitamins, trace mineral formulas, and specific minerals such as calcium or magnesium.

The following agents help to eliminate biofilm:

- Biofilm-busting enzymes: The following enzymes help digest and break down biofilm:
  - Serrapeptase: 40,000 to 60,000 U per day, away from food.

- Nattokinase (derived from natto, a fermented soy product): 20,000 FU two to three times per day, away from food.
- Lumbrokinase: an enzyme derived from a type of earthworm. Its activity is about ten times that of nattokinase, but it is also significantly more expensive. The brand Boluoke has the best research behind it. Take one capsule two times per day, away from food (600,000 U per day total).

- InterFase Plus: this product contains enzymes with the addition of disodium EDTA (ethylenediaminetetraacetic acid) and chitosans that also help break down biofilm. Take one to two capsules twice a day between meals.

- Lactoferrin: This molecule binds up iron, which effectively prevents the formation of biofilm. Be careful using this if you are already iron-deficient or anemic. Do not take it if you have a dairy allergy, as it is derived from dairy and could worsen your symptoms. Consult with your healthcare provider to determine if it is safe for you to use. Take 600 milligrams one to two times per day.

- Xylitol: This low-carbohydrate sweetener is naturally found in low amounts in some fruits and vegetables. Even though it is as sweet as table sugar, it has 40 percent fewer calories and does not cause an increase in blood sugar, so it is safe for diabetics. It has been shown to make the biofilm weaker in dental studies. Although it is safe for humans, it is extremely toxic to dogs, so avoid keeping it around your pets. Take 1 teaspoon three to four times a day in water or juice to start, and you can increase to up to 1 tablespoon three to four times a day. Some people get gas and bloating with xylitol, so you may have to ramp up your dose slowly.

- Coconut oil (organic): Coconut oil has been used to treat various infections, including bacterial and yeast infections, and contains the compound monolaurin, which disrupts biofilm formation. Take 1 tablespoon twice a day with food.
- *N*-acetylcysteine (NAC): This amino acid has been used to help break up mucus in the body and has been shown in numerous studies to break up biofilm. Take 200 to 600 milligrams three times per day. NAC may deplete zinc and copper when used long-term, so I recommend supplementing with these minerals if you take NAC for more than two months. NAC can cause gastrointestinal distress in some individuals and should not be taken by anyone with an active stomach ulcer.

I do not recommend taking all of the suggested products simultaneously. To follow my standard protocol, please take serrapeptase, InterFase Plus, and NAC (as recommended in the preceding list). I often have people add coconut oil into their cooking instead of taking additional supplements. The other supplements may be appropriate for you if you cannot tolerate or are allergic to one of the other products listed. You have options to consider if you need to find another way to break down biofilm.

What More Can I Do?

In addition to following the Lyme-specific protocol and busting biofilms, to overcome Lyme disease you must support your immune system. The immune system is complex, but to grasp the basics, think of it in two parts. The first parts of the immune system consist of cells (T-cytotoxic and natural killer, or NK, cells) that identify foreign microbes and begin to eliminate them right away. The second part of the immune system consists of the cells (called T helper cells) that stimulate specific antibodies in response to foreign microbes. The goal is to strengthen part one—that is, to increase the number of direct scavenger cells that can quickly identify an invading organism and eradicate it as soon as possible. It's not usually necessary to increase the number of antibody-producing cells, as this may trigger the inflammatory autoimmune response. The herbs and nutrients that can help keep the first part of your immune system active and healthy include:

- Vitamin C. Numerous studies show that vitamin C helps with active infections and may help improve the effect of antibiotics. Test-tube studies show that large doses of vitamin C may inhibit the growth of bacteria or kill it altogether. Take 1,000 milligrams two to three times per day. You can increase the dose up to 2,000 milligrams three times per day if tolerated. High doses of vitamin C can cause abdominal pain or loose stool, so reduce the dose if this occurs. Vitamin C also increases the absorption of iron, so do not use it if you are genetically predisposed to iron overload. A simple blood test can ensure that you are not storing too much iron.
- Vitamin D. I find that 90 percent of the people with Lyme who consult me have deficient or low-normal blood levels of vitamin D. In the United States, vitamin D deficiency affects more than 40 percent of people.[16] The best way to get vitamin D is through sunlight exposure without sunblock. Cod liver oil is the highest food source of vitamin D, with about 1,300

IU in 1 tablespoon. Eggs, dairy products, and some fish contain smaller amounts. Because of concerns about skin cancer,
when outdoors for an extended time, most people wear long
clothing or sunscreen. But this effectively blocks the absorption of UV radiation, which is necessary to make vitamin D
naturally. Try to get twenty to thirty minutes of unblocked
sun exposure daily during the nonpeak sun hours such as before eleven a.m. or after four p.m. to help increase your vitamin D levels. In this way, you can meet your vitamin D needs
while also avoiding skin aging through the sun's UV radiation.
If this is not possible or you live in a cold climate, take 2,000
to 4,000 IU of supplemental vitamin D3 per day with food.

Vitamin D Toxicity

Most health-care providers can periodically test your vitamin D blood
levels to ensure that you take the optimal dose. Blood vitamin D
levels should be over 50 ng/mL. Blood levels greater than 100 ng/mL
may signify toxicity, so reduce your vitamin D intake if your blood
level gets too high. Signs of vitamin D toxicity include loss of appetite, weight loss, heart palpitations, and elevated blood calcium. Although at excessive doses vitamin D can be toxic, I have never seen
vitamin D toxicity in clinical practice, even when people take high
doses of supplemental vitamin D. You would likely have to take more
than 10,000 IU daily for many weeks to months to reach toxic levels,
and most people just don't supplement with that much vitamin D.
Nonetheless, I advise you to check your blood levels to make sure
you are getting the correct amount.

- Zinc, an immune stimulator, contributes to many metabolic
  bodily processes. It is an effective antiviral and anti-

inflammatory nutrient. Zinc deficiency is a widely unrecognized nutritional deficiency and may affect up to two billion people worldwide.[17] Signs of zinc deficiency can include:

- Loss of smell or taste
- Getting sick often
- Acne
- Eczema
- Poor wound healing
- Diarrhea
- Mouth ulcers
- Anorexia
- Behavior problems
- Depression or attention-deficit disorder
- Horizontal white spots in the fingernails

This is yet another reason that following *The Lyme Solution* diet is so important. The most common cause of zinc deficiency is inadequate dietary intake. Most processed foods are deficient in or completely depleted of zinc. I recommend taking 30 to 50 milligrams per day with food. Take zinc with food, as it can nauseate you if taken on an empty stomach. Long-term use of zinc supplements can induce a deficiency of folate or copper. Taking a high-quality multivitamin can offset that deficiency.

- Andrographis. *Andrographis paniculata*, a potent antimicrobial and anti-inflammatory herb native to India, China, and other Southeast Asian countries, has been used for centuries to treat various infections. More recently, doctors are finding it effective in treating rheumatoid arthritis and ulcerative colitis.[18] Research shows that andrographis helps increase the output of molecules in the gut lining and other mucous membranes that directly attack bacteria. These molecules, called *defensins*, are part of our first line of defense against invading microbes.

You can find andrographis in many forms, but I prefer an encapsulated standardized extract. Take 300 to 400 milligrams twice a day of a 50 percent andrographolide product.

Putting It All Together

When I started Lyme treatment myself, I had no idea that I was in for a wild ride. The day-to-day ups and downs of feeling better and then worse can start to wear you out physically and emotionally. Now that I am on the back end of treatment and have treated so many other people with Lyme disease, I see that the Lyme roller coaster is normal. As much as I would like to see continual progress, that is rare. You'll go through stretches where your energy and joint pain feel better. On other days you can barely crawl out of bed or function. It's the nature of the shape-shifter. You just need to find the right way to tame it.

Following both *The Lyme Solution* diet as well as using the recommended herbal protocols will help to reduce your bodily load of Lyme disease. Breaking up the biofilm will allow the herbs to work more efficiently. If you start to get a lot of herxing, use the anti-inflammatory and detoxifying herbs more. The herxing will pass. Keep your immune system primed with the nutrients and herbs that support it best. You will often feel like you're constantly choking down a bunch of pills or liquids. Yes, it can take a bit of organization to stay on task, but it's worth it. When you start to have more good days than bad days, you're on your way to recovery.

CHAPTER 6

Hidden Toxins in Your Surroundings

Over the years, I've worked with many people who have taken antibiotics or herbs to treat their Lyme disease but still struggle with some of their symptoms. While reducing the body load of microbes can improve your health significantly, sometimes killing the bugs is not enough. In this chapter, I'll offer ways to address a broader spectrum of factors that can undermine your health.

An All-Encompassing Disruption

Since few conventional doctors tally all of the harmful factors that can undermine the immune system, you may be astounded at the myriad ways your lifestyle and surroundings challenge your body's capacity to recover from Lyme disease. The conventional medicine approach to health is based on the presumption that your body exists on its own, in some pristine environment, like a laboratory. After all, that is where microbes are studied! Obviously, that is not the case. The human organism lives in a constant interaction with its environment, and what's going on in our homes, workplaces, communities, and society cannot help but affect us. Yet most health care fails to take that interaction into account. As a result, conventional medicine provides no tools for assessing or dealing with harmful factors in our surroundings.

For example, since you began to experience Lyme disease symptoms, have you noticed any difference in your reaction to chemicals or odors? Are your seasonal allergies worse? Do you feel that you get sick more than other people around you? Are you feeling more sluggish and less motivated than you used to? Countless people report these and other changes. But no one tells people the reason why—that when you have Lyme disease, your body and immune system have undergone an all-encompassing alteration. The disruption can leave you with an oversensitive body that reacts to a wide range of toxic triggers that you never noticed before. Although you may be able to avoid some irritants like cigarette smoke or scented candles, other allergens or toxins, such as mold, can be difficult to escape.

Fortunately, there is a subspecialty in medicine called *environmental medicine* that assesses and accounts for the toxic outputs released into our world that we end up absorbing. Environmental medicine also seeks greater understanding of how those outputs affect us.

When It Comes to Toxins, the Body Is Like a Barrel

Environmental medicine doctors sometimes characterize the body as a barrel. While there is no literal barrel in your body, this metaphor reminds us that every single one of us has physiological limits, something medicine rarely mentions. If you keep absorbing toxins and fail to release them, then at some point the barrel gets full and overflows. And when your barrel overflows, you become sicker and sicker. You start to feel tired, your body aches, you have difficulty concentrating, and you have constipation or diarrhea, bad breath, heartburn, sleep problems, skin rashes or eczema, sinus congestion, constant runny nose, or headaches.

Until that happens and symptoms show up, the average person won't know how close they are to the point where enough is enough. Some people are born with a large barrel and others with a shot glass. In other words, both the capacity to tolerate and the capacity to release toxins are unique for each individual. Moreover, people live in different surroundings, in differing dwellings, and in various degrees of proximity to the toxic outputs of industry and agriculture. All of these contribute to the load in your barrel. Although the barrel and the load are metaphors, they describe actual biological processes going on in everyone's body. I learned to apply these concepts to my medical practice when I studied with and was mentored by Bill Rea, MD, of the Environmental Health Center in Dallas, Texas. One of the forefathers of environmental medicine, Dr. Rea has written a four-volume textbook for physicians (*Chemical Sensitivity*) on how to identify and reduce toxic load in the body. He has treated more than thirty thousand patients over a fifty-year medical career. Along with me, he has educated thousands of other physicians around the world in how to find and address the hidden causes of disease through understanding toxicity.

Based on this view, to maintain or recover your health requires two things: First, limit harmful activities and toxic exposures in order to keep your barrel from filling up and overflowing. Second, pay attention to specific features of your surroundings: your chemical exposure, your sleep patterns, your exercise regimen, and the sources of stress that affect your barrel. In this chapter, you will learn how to ease the toxic burden on your body by avoiding toxins through making the right lifestyle changes as well as cleaning up your surroundings. Chapter 7 takes a thorough look at how to get healing sleep and gentle exercise, and at other tools, like meditation, that will help prevent the damaging effects of stress.

First of all, I recommend decreasing your body burden of dangerous toxins by replacing items you use daily in your home with natural, nontoxic products. Taking these simple measures to reduce your exposure to harmful chemicals will make it easier for your body to detoxify. The result is that your immune system will function better. I am also going to show you how to look for potentially toxic mold, which can cause Lyme-like symptoms, that may be lurking in your home. Making your home a safe haven, free from toxic chemicals and mold, gives your body the best chance to get well.

ELLIE'S STORY

I met Ellie several years after she had originally been diagnosed with Lyme disease. She was one of the lucky ones who found her Lyme disease right away and was treated early, so she was no longer having many of the symptoms she had when she first became sick. However, she recently started having daily headaches and brain fog. Ellie worked as a music therapist in a nursing home. Often forgetful at work, she had difficulty remembering the names of some of the patients with whom she was working.

Ellie was eating well, exercised regularly, and had a low-stress life. There was nothing in her life that could explain why all of a sudden she was feeling unwell. I started her on some herbs and nutrients to give her symptomatic relief but knew we hadn't gotten to the cause of her illness. I asked her if anything had changed at work—new construction, new furniture, or fresh paint. She didn't think so, but when she asked her boss, he told her they had recently installed air fresheners throughout the entire facility. The air fresheners were hidden out of sight, so Ellie had no idea that while she was at work all day, she was exposed to the wide array of chemicals the air fresheners released into the air she breathed.

Suspecting that this was causing her headaches and brain fog, I suggested she take some time off to get out of the office. After a week of being away, her headaches were gone and her brain fog lifted. It was now clear that even though she was not able to smell the fragrance, the air fresheners were making her sick. When Ellie discussed this with her boss, he agreed to have them removed in her work area, and her symptoms disappeared. Some people are more sensitive than others. For them, even a little bit of exposure to a toxic chemical can cause big health problems. Avoiding chemicals whenever you can gives you the best chance to get well.

Going Chemical-Free

Making lifestyle changes can be difficult. I make it a core feature of my Five-Stage Immune-Boosting Plan, because for countless people, making these changes spells the difference between success and failure in resolving Lyme disease.

The world is filled with numerous toxins and toxicants that adversely affect health. (Toxins come from plants and animals, while toxicants are specifically human-made or artificial products.) Getting chemicals out of your home, work, and school environment may be one of the most important things you can do for your health. It is also the simplest.

It's always a good idea—and absolutely critical when you have an immune system challenge like Lyme disease—to remove from your surroundings as many toxins and toxicants as you can. Even if you do nothing else, this will automatically lessen the load of poisons that make you sick. You may not have shut the faucet off completely, but you can reduce it to a manageable drip.

Where to begin? Become aware of your immediate surroundings within your home and workplace. Instead of accepting that a load of toxic chemicals is just part of modern life, start paying attention to what's in your house, car, and workspace. Next, notice what you eat, apply to your body, use, and wear. The next step is getting rid of all you can of the following:

- Air fresheners
- Cleaning chemicals
- Detergents
- Disinfectants
- Plastic water bottles
- Lawn-care products, including Roundup
- Lead-based dishes, glasses, or pottery
- Petrochemical products, such as turpentine
- Pressed-board furniture (MDF—medium-density fiber-board)
- Scented candles
- Wall-to-wall carpet (numerous chemicals saturate new carpet, while old carpet tends to be moldy)

These products all contain dangerous compounds that can significantly increase the toxic burden on your body. Many of these products contain petroleum, toluene, benzene, and other chemicals that have been associated with causing cancer, asthma, allergies, and other health issues.[1] All of them have the potential to alter or suppress your immune system, making it more difficult to fight off infection.[2]

PRODUCT SUBSTITUTION CHART

STOP USING . . .	START USING . . .
Tub and tile cleaners containing ammonia, bleach, artificial fragrances, detergents, or aerosolized propellants	Baking soda in warm water or a nonchlorinated scouring powder, such as Bon Ami
Mold or mildew cleaners containing formaldehyde, phenol, kerosene, or pentachlorophenol	Borax or distilled vinegar in hot water
Glass cleaners with ammonia and dye	Rubbing alcohol
Disinfectants with cresol, phenol, formaldehyde, ammonia, or chlorine	Soap and warm water
Dry cleaners that use perchloroethylene (perc) or trichlorethylene	Wear clothes that do not require dry cleaning or find an organic cleaner in your area that uses nontoxic cleaners
Laundry detergents with artificial fragrances, dyes, chlorine, or synthetic whiteners	Fragrance-free, dye-free organic laundry detergents
Air fresheners that contain naphthalene, phenol, cresol, ethanol, xylene, or formaldehyde	Box of baking soda or bag of silica gel to help remove odors; use natural fragrances or essential oils in a diffuser to scent the air
Paint with volatile organic compounds (VOCs)	VOC-free paint

STOP USING . . .	START USING . . .
Shampoos and soaps with fragrances, artificial colors, detergents, cresol or polyvinylpyrrolidone (PVP) plastics. There are many toxic chemicals in these products, so if you can't pronounce it, don't buy it!	Castile soap or other fragrance-free, dye-free shampoo or body wash
Toothpaste and mouthwash (especially with fluoride)	Fluoride-free toothpaste with no artificial coloring or flavors
Cosmetics with artificial fragrances, colors, PVP, mineral oil, talc, or alcohol	Natural cosmetics, free of these chemicals
Deodorant with antiperspirant that contains aluminum	Natural deodorant
Sunscreen with parabens or artificial fragrances	Wear protective clothing or use natural sunscreen that is paraben-free
Pesticides and herbicides	Use natural pyrethrins from chrysanthemum and organic fertilizers
Insect repellents with DEET	Herbal insect repellents with essential oils

Outgassing

You should consider any new products in your home potentially toxic. Why? The chemicals they contain will be released into the air (known as *outgassing*) over many weeks and months. Be careful with new furniture, paint, clothing, and any other item that you bring inside. I recommend that you buy furniture made from nontoxic materials (including nontoxic wood), metal, glass, or organic fiber to eliminate the possibility of breathing in toxic gases.

Furniture coverings, for example, may contain chemicals to preserve (or fire-proof) the fabric and wood. If you have already purchased new furniture, that "new" smell means that it may contain toxic chemicals. Put it in a garage (or another room you don't use much) to allow it to outgas until the odor is completely gone. If you need to paint or repaint your home, use low- or no-VOC paints that limit your exposure to formaldehyde and phenol. New clothing should always be washed before wearing to get rid of the formaldehyde. You may even need to wash articles of clothing two to three times to get the chemicals out completely. If the clothes still have an odor after washing and drying them, throw them back in for another cycle.

One of the biggest sources of toxic exposures is a new car. That "new-car smell" is literally the outgassing of toxic chemicals such as formaldehyde, phenol, polyvinyl chloride (PVC), flame retardants, adhesives, glues, and lubricants. Dozens of chemicals are released inside the car that can take months to years to completely outgas. I recommend buying a car that is at least two years old, so that your exposure to these noxious chemicals is drastically reduced. If you happen to own a new car, the best way to expedite the outgassing is to "bake" the car. Get it out in the sun with the windows or sunroof open. The heat will help to get the chemicals out. Although it is not a quick process, it can definitely shorten the time to make your car less toxic. You can also put a box of baking soda in the car to help absorb some of the chemicals in the interior.

Personal-Care Products

Many are surprised to learn that the personal-care products we rely on to clean and beautify ourselves actually contain numerous toxic chemicals. From daily use of the following, we receive frequent toxic inputs:

- Antiperspirants and deodorants
- Cologne
- Conditioners
- Hair dye
- Hair spray, gel, or mousse
- Lotions
- Makeup
- Nail polish and polish remover
- Perfume
- Shampoos
- Soaps
- Sunscreen

Product ingredients such as parabens, sodium lauryl sulfate, petroleum, and aluminum not only are common allergens but also disrupt the hormones and immune system.[3] Doctors call these chemicals *endocrine disruptors*, since they alter the way hormones normally work. Yet most people use these products every day on their hair and skin. The result? The number of chemicals that can steadily accumulate in your body is strikingly high.[4] And what is most frightening is the effect of these chemicals on pregnant moms and their babies. Since most of these toxic chemicals are stored in fat cells and organs, a pregnant mother is at a higher risk for storing them, since fat mass increases during pregnancy and the toxins have more places to hide.

These seemingly safe everyday products you use in your home or on your skin can have devastating effects on the baby, both in the womb and after delivery. If a mom has extensive exposure to these chemicals during her pregnancy, the baby can be born with chronic immune problems, developmental delays, and an inability to process toxins on his or her own.[5] Recent research into the adverse effects of plasticizers like bisphenol A (BPA) and phthalates reveals their dangers. They are found in food and drink packaging (plastic water bottles), the lining of cans of food, compact discs, plastic toys, and some medical devices. Persistent exposure to these chemicals can lead to early onset of puberty in children, hormone disruption in people of both sexes, reproductive and genital defects in newborns, and low testosterone or sperm count in males.[6]

This makes me wonder how much early exposure to these chemicals affects the immune system over the long term. Unfortunately, there are no good studies of the cumulative effect of the thousands of chemicals we are exposed to each year that might reveal more about their impact on the immune system. The safest thing is to avoid as many of these toxins as possible to keep your risk to the bare minimum.

Your Home, Yard, and Community

In addition to personal-care products, you need to exercise caution with outdoor chemicals such as pesticides and herbicides. Once applied to your lawn or plants, they can stay in the ground for decades. Every year these chemicals are reapplied—since they are added more rapidly than they break down—the soil content of endangering toxins increases. Of the more than 84,000 chemicals used in the United States today, only about 200 of them have ever been studied for their long-term safety as required by the Environmental Protection Agency (EPA).[7]

What this means is the stuff you use outdoors can be just as toxic as what you use indoors. One of the most popular U.S. pesticides is Roundup, which is used in lawn-care products as well as in agriculture. Roundup's main ingredient is a compound called glyphosate, which the World Health Organization has recently stated likely causes cancer.[8] Additionally, glyphosate may also alter immune function toward autoimmunity and create more inflammation.[9] Dr. Gilles-Éric Séralini, a French molecular biologist, found in his research that the "inactive" ingredients in Roundup are more than a thousand times as toxic as glyphosate.[10] And yet companies that make these herbicides are not required to study the potential toxic effects on humans of these inactive ingredients, which are automatically deemed safe. There is plenty of good evidence that these chemicals are not safe at any level and should be avoided for your own health and the health of your family.

Your Town or City

Anyone fighting an immune system challenge must take a closer look at the toxins released into their immediate town or city and region. The list of communities that have become dangerously polluted grows longer every year. Toxic exposures often cause major health issues. One example is the case of hexavalent chromium contamination in the water supply of Hinkley, California. This deadly chemical, used for preventing corrosion in their tanks, made hundreds of town residents ill (and was the basis of the movie *Erin Brockovich*).

In another recent incident, tap water in Flint, Michigan, was found to be contaminated with toxic levels of lead. After the city switched its water source from Lake Huron to the Flint River in 2014, the more corrosive river water began leaching lead from the city's century-old water pipes into the city water system, making many residents very sick. Lead is toxic to the brain and nervous system and can lead to headaches, numbness in arms and legs, poor appetite, poor focus or concentration, memory loss, lower IQ, growth delays in children, behavior changes, and abdominal pain. As you can see, many poisonous toxicants from industry cannot be so readily avoided. That makes it even more essential to avoid exposure to the ones that you can.

Unfortunately, there is no easy way to measure the load of toxic chemicals within your body, nor to determine specifically how they affect your health. While billions of dollars are spent testing pricey pharmaceuticals, too little research assesses the health risks of toxic chemicals. But if you want to recover your immune system and your health, you cannot afford to wait around for the full scientific proof. There is enough evidence now to take action.

Reduce or eliminate entirely your exposure to toxic personal-care products, cleaning supplies, and lawn-care products. One of my favorite books, *Toxic Free* by Debra Lynn Dadd, gives you natural alternatives to many conventional cleaning products commonly used around the house. You'll find a lot of chemical-free items at your local health food store as well. Check out the Campaign for Safer Cosmetics (safecosmetics.org) for information on what to look for in shopping for personal-care products. You can also go to Safer Chemicals, Healthy Families (saferchemicals.org) to ask for better research and safety regulations on toxic chemicals. The Environmental Working Group (ewg.org) can also show you which products are safer to use and less likely to adversely affect your immune system.

Mold: The Unwanted Guest That's Making You Sick

Because it resembles so many other illnesses, Lyme disease is known as "the Great Imitator." And nothing looks more like Lyme disease than toxic-mold exposure. The symptoms of Lyme disease and symptoms of mold exposure are almost identical. Even the blood tests doctors like me run for various immune and inflammatory markers are similar. What makes mold particularly difficult and potentially dangerous is that most people who have mold in their immediate surroundings are not aware that they have been or are currently being exposed. Small leaks in your roof, bathroom, kitchen, or walls can go undetected for months or years and trigger chronic health issues. Don't assume that, because you don't see any water damage, there is none. I am always suspicious when someone tells me that their symptoms improve when they're away from home, or away from some other place they frequent, such as a school or a workplace.

You can find molds, which are types of fungi, just about everywhere, but they particularly like areas with a lot of moisture. Moisture is necessary for mold growth. This is why water-damaged buildings can be so dangerous: wet materials like wood, insulation, or drywall provide an optimal environment for the mold to continue growing. Mold often hides behind walls or under cabinets or appliances and other areas that are difficult to see. Some people can smell mold when they walk into a building, but just because you can't smell it, that doesn't mean it isn't there.

Do your own home inspection. Check under cabinets, particularly wherever there is a sink or water source. If you have an attic or basement, look for signs of a leak or stagnant water. Water staining on wood or drywall is a sign of a leak and should be investigated. Bathrooms and kitchens are common places for water damage, since there are water sources going in and out of these rooms. Mold can look black, gray, tan, green, or yellow and has a velvety, fuzzy appearance. You will often see water stains under or around where the mold is growing. As you do your inspection, wear a painter's mask and gloves to minimize your exposure.

Aside from mold exposure from leaky roofs and appliances, mold in food can be another source of contamination. Some foods are intentionally moldy, such as aged cheeses, like blue cheese or Stilton cheese, or mushrooms. People who are allergic to mold in the air are often also allergic to mold in cheese, which can cause a similar allergic reaction. Mold can also get into other foods by accident. Dried fruits or fruit juices, smoked meats, many canned foods, vinegar, condiments, and fermented foods like sauerkraut tend to have mold in them and can be problematic for individuals with Lyme. Peanuts are known to contain a specific type of mycotoxin called aflatoxin, which is associated with causing liver cancer, autoimmune illness, and even death. Mold can also get into leftover foods. Any food not consumed within twenty-four hours of cooking should be either frozen or discarded. The likelihood of mold contamination goes up the longer it sits in the fridge. Do not try to cut off the moldy part of a food and eat the rest. Mold spores are microscopic, so the non-moldy-looking part of the food may still have mold in it. I advise anyone with Lyme to be aware of moldy foods and to avoid them when possible.

ANNE'S STORY

Anne is a typical Type A personality, always on the go with a very hectic lifestyle. Several years ago, when she started to become fatigued, she figured she was just working too hard and needed more rest. She cut her schedule back and worked from home more often, but instead of feeling better, she found her symptoms worsening. She now experienced headaches, brain fog, dizziness, and muscle weakness.

I ran several blood tests, including tests for Lyme. Her Lyme test was negative, but her inflammatory markers were elevated. Although I still suspected that Lyme played a role in her health issues, I was concerned that other problems were making her sick.

Anne lived in an old home near the beach in California. Although she had never had her home tested for mold, there had been a leak under her sink for many months. When she had a professional inspection done, they found very high levels of mold, including the very toxic *Stachybotrys*. This is one of the more common toxic molds found in water-damaged buildings and is linked with numerous health issues. It produces several types of mycotoxins that are dangerous when inhaled. I advised Anne to move out while she had her house remediated. Within a week of being out of her house, her symptoms started to improve. The longer she stayed away, the better she felt. Her plan to kick back and work more from home was making her more toxic and sick! I started her on a protocol to get rid of mold toxins in her body. This included sweating out the toxins with regular exercise, binding up the toxins in her gut with bentonite clay, and doing regular saunas at her local gym. After three months of treatment, she was symptom-free.

The microscopic spores that mold releases into the air are what make mold a health hazard. Once you inhale these mold spores, two issues ensue. First, many molds produce toxic chemicals called mycotoxins, which can directly damage the nervous system and lungs. Second, mold spores can trigger an allergic reaction that affects your brain, lungs, gut, and other organs. This combination of mold toxicity and allergy can create a cluster of symptoms that look and feel like Lyme disease.

A well-known cases of mold toxicity occurred in the home of former *Tonight Show* sidekick Ed McMahon and his wife, Pamela. A ruptured pipe and botched repair led to a buildup of *Stachybotrys* in their home, and both became very ill. The McMahons eventually had to move out of their home until the work was completed correctly.

Mold spores are found everywhere, but not everyone gets sick just because they are exposed to mold. However, I find people with Lyme disease seem to have a special sensitivity to mold and should take appropriate measures to minimize their exposure.

Kelly McCann, MD, of Costa Mesa, California, one of the foremost experts on mold and mycotoxins, notes that they can cause a chronic inflammatory reaction that affects the brain, causing fatigue, mood changes, depression, stress, and sleep disruption.[11] Mycotoxins can also cause your immune system to form antibodies that react to your own nervous system. This autoimmune reaction can dull your senses. It can make it more difficult to walk and maintain balance and coordination. Exposure to certain molds may also lead to the following:

- Poor regulation of heart rate, breathing, sweating, coordination, and hormone balance
- Joint or muscle pain
- Body stiffness
- Blurry vision
- Dizziness
- Persistent cough
- Headaches
- Numbness or tingling in skin
- Night sweats
- Changes with urination

Note that all of these symptoms are also present in Lyme disease. If you have these symptoms, it's easy to conclude that you have Lyme disease—but it's not necessarily so. Anyone with these or other Lyme-like symptoms should be evaluated for mold toxicity or allergy. You should also have your home tested by a professional mold inspector—even if you are not sure if there has been a leak.

Testing for Mold

While there are many ways to test for mold, hire a company that uses one of three primary methods:

1. Spore trap sampling. The spore trapping machine sucks in air and traps it onto a sticky surface, which is then cultured in a lab for mold spores. The lab also analyzes a sample collected from outside the home as a baseline to compare to your indoor mold counts.

2. Direct mold sampling. This method takes samples in areas with visible water damage or mold growth and cultures the samples in a lab. The result is a direct measurement of what is growing on the damaged surface.

3. Environmental Relative Moldiness Index (ERMI). This new technique measures the type and amount of mold present in your home's dust. It is often used as a screening tool, since a single dust sample may not capture the total mold load in the home. ERMI studies the DNA of thirty-six different mold species known to cause health issues. The scale ranges from −10 to 20, but any score over 5 suggests that your home is in the highest 25 percent of homes with the greatest mold burden. The higher the number, the greater the likelihood of mold issues. If the ERMI score is greater than 5, then you should do spore trap sampling to get

more specific information about the type and amounts of mold in your home.

Home Testing for Mold

You can also test your home with petri dishes available from many home improvement stores. You leave the open petri dishes in the room being tested for up to four hours, then seal the plates and send them to the lab for testing. While this method is very inexpensive, it is not as accurate as having a professional company measure mold in your home. This method will detect only what is floating in the air at the time you collect the sample and does not necessarily represent what's in the room over a longer period of time. Mold does not release its spores at a constant rate, so it's possible to miss the window when the spores are at their peak when you do the test.

Keep in mind, though, that many people who have gotten a negative result after doing their own home testing later find after professional testing that they had very high levels of mold in their home. Home testing with a petri dish is a good screening tool for a reasonable price. Just be aware that false negatives are common. If your plate testing comes back negative and you are still suspicious of mold in your home, it's worth paying a good company to give you more accurate information.

If you do discover that you have high levels of mold, consult with a mold remediation specialist to find the best way to get rid of it. Be aware that most general contractors are not mold specialists and do not have expertise in remediating mold correctly. Unfortunately, mold remediation can be costly, depending on the extent of the damage. But a prolonged illness can be far more costly, on many levels.

How to Prevent Indoor Mold

A lot of mold spores originate outdoors—there's little you can do about them. But here are tips to keep mold from growing in your home:

- Remove all carpet. Both the carpet and the padding underneath can trap mold spores. If the carpet has ever been steam cleaned, there is a chance that mold is growing on the subfloor. It is very difficult to remove all of the water once the carpet has been cleaned. Replace the carpet with wood, tile, or ceramic floors. Mold cannot grow as easily on hard surfaces. Put a throw rug over the hard surface for comfort—these are much easier to clean than wall-to-wall carpet.

- Use a high-quality HEPA filter in your home. These filters can remove mold spores, dust, pollen, and other particulates floating in the air. Depending on the size of the HEPA filter, you may need to use more than one. I recommend using one in the bedroom and one in a room that you spend most of your time in other than sleeping. Some high-quality air filters also come with a carbon filter than can remove chemicals from the air, which is helpful if you are also chemically sensitive. I do not recommend air filters that emit ozone, as ozone can be irritating to your nose and lungs.

- Use a dehumidifier if you have a basement or live in a high-humidity part of the world. This will keep the moisture inside the home at a safe level so that mold does not easily grow. Keep your indoor humidity between 40 and 50 percent. Many dehumidifiers can be set to a desired humidity.

- Keep windows closed in the evenings and overnight if you are allergic or sensitive to mold. Most mold sporulation occurs in the early evening. Open windows at that time invite those mold spores, which can trigger symptoms, into your home.

Exposure to mycotoxins, toxins from fungi, is dangerous because they directly damage your nervous system and lungs, which can be extensive and lethal. Most people who have been exposed and have thereby developed mycotoxicity don't know it, because mold testing does not measure mycotoxins. And even though some molds, such as *Stachybotrys* or chaetomium, are known to produce mycotoxins, it doesn't necessarily mean that they have done so. If you find high levels of toxic molds in your home, you will need to work with your doctor to have other tests done to see if you also have mycotoxicity. For some people, I order a urine test by Real Time Labs that measures for four types of mycotoxins. This gives me a good idea of whether someone has had exposure. It is an expensive test but can help you figure out if mycotoxins are part of your total body burden of toxins.

While exposure to mycotoxins from mold is more dangerous, the more common issue is mold allergy. Most of the people I work with who have Lyme disease are allergic to mold and feel worse on damp, rainy, or humid days when outdoor mold counts escalate. They will often feel ill when they are in a moldy building or damp basement. Some individuals with Lyme who get very ill when they are in moldy environments have no evidence of mycotoxicity. This leads me to believe that mold allergy is the larger issue for them. I suspect that their immune reaction to mold produces antibodies that cause inflammation in the brain, resulting in many neurological symptoms. I will talk more in Chapter 8 about how to treat your mold allergy and reduce your body burden.

. . . .

CHAPTER 7

More Sleep, More Exercise, Less Stress

In working with people with Lyme disease, I am both counselor and physician. In these dual roles, I have seen time and again how much chronic illness stresses the person who has it, along with his or her loved ones and anyone who serves as a caregiver. People with Lyme disease can easily become overwhelmed when they don't feel well. It's a challenge to manage all the therapies they use to recover their health. Some people can't go to school or work or participate in activities they count on to bring joy to their lives. It's no wonder so many feel frustrated and sad.

I have also seen people coping with Lyme become isolated from their friends and family. If you're in this situation, you might become concerned that your friends and loved ones have grown weary of hearing the details of your illness. You might at times feel that you are the only one in the world dealing with it—but you're not. Millions of others like you struggle with the symptoms that plague you each day. For many, Lyme disease is a daily reminder of how painful it can be to lose the things that they treasure and the life they once lived. Being able to stay centered on this emotional roller coaster can be very stressful. That is why it is so important to develop the tools for doing so.

When you are unwell, you need to give yourself permission to do whatever is required for your recovery. Your health needs to be a priority. If you are the caretaker of the family, you cannot easily fill that role if you aren't well. Many people with Lyme feel guilty for taking time to heal, but it is important to give your body the tools it needs to allow the healing process to happen—whether it's going to an exercise class, taking ten minutes out of your day to meditate, or making a commitment to get to bed earlier. It's perfectly okay to take care of yourself, so don't beat yourself up for making the commitment to better health.

Sleep: The Time to Repair and Restore

A good night's sleep is the foundation for the resilience you need to recover. Yet many complain that they have trouble sleeping through the night or sleeping deeply. Sleep deprivation leads to further fatigue, brain fog, poor memory, poor concentration, and irritability. If you investigate the sleep patterns of different cultures, you'll be surprised to find out that bedtime varies. So does how long people sleep. You would think that as humans, all people would have the same sleep requirements and sleep on a relatively similar schedule. Not so. The amount of sleep you need and get depends on different factors: age, physical health, stress, medications, the sleeping environment, and diet. With so many variables that affect the quality and quantity of sleep, experts disagree about the best time to go to bed and how long you should sleep. However, they all agree that those who don't get deep sleep both die younger and experience more chronic health issues—including obesity, increased risk for heart attack, and less brainpower. It is during deep sleep that your body repairs and restores itself. What goes on when you sleep? From a physiological perspective, sleep is complex and involves several hormones and neurotransmitters. To get a good night's sleep, all of them need to be working properly.

The process of sleep requires a well-orchestrated balance of hormones and brain chemicals (called *neurotransmitters*) all playing their parts to help you fall asleep, stay asleep, and wake up feeling refreshed. The body follows a twenty-four-hour clock that responds to light and darkness, called a *circadian rhythm*, that controls sleep, hormone release, body temperature, and other normal body functions. It is often referred to as our *biological clock*. If the circadian rhythm gets disrupted, it can lead to obesity, diabetes, depression, bipolar disorder, and seasonal affective disorder.[1]

Stimulating neurotransmitters, such as dopamine, epinephrine, norepinephrine, glutamate, and histamine, keep you awake. Other neurotransmitters with the opposite effect help you fall asleep. These include gamma-aminobutyric acid (GABA) and serotonin. While most people think of neurotransmitters as either stimulating or sedating, most neurotransmitters actually do both. Cytokines, immune chemicals that get released during an infection, are another powerful influence on sleep. This is why so many people feel tired when they are sick—their immune system is trying to fight the infection.

The neurotransmitter melatonin regulates the sleep cycle and helps people fall asleep. In the pineal gland, melatonin is converted from serotonin. As melatonin levels rise, you become drowsy and your body temperature drops—one reason people feel colder at bedtime. Since melatonin is inhibited by light, using an iPad or smartphone before bedtime may interfere with sleep, tricking your brain into responding as if it were still daytime. Many people with Lyme find that their biggest issue is *falling* asleep. Others say they wake several times in the night. Occasionally, it's both issues.

Cortisol, a hormone secreted by the adrenal glands, rises about twenty minutes before you wake up. Cortisol has many functions in the body, but one of its jobs is to increase our blood sugar. So if your last meal was early in the evening and you haven't had any food in eight to ten hours and your blood sugar starts to drop, cortisol is released to help increase your blood sugar and keep it balanced. Since cortisol is also a major stress hormone, when you are under a lot of stress, your cortisol levels mount. If your stress goes on for months or years, your cortisol can start to drop and your ability to control stress, blood sugar, energy, and sleep can all be abnormally affected.

No matter what time you go to bed, sleep occurs in 90- to 120-minute cycles, which consist of deep, non-REM sleep followed by lighter REM sleep. As the night progresses, the ratio of deep to light sleep shifts, so that you spend more time in REM sleep in the few hours before waking. REM (rapid eye movement) sleep occurs 70 to 90 minutes after you fall asleep, and it is during this time of your sleep cycle that your brain and body are able to repair and restore themselves. We dream while in REM sleep, which is why most people remember their dreams right before they wake. People who go to bed later in the night may also miss more time in deep, restorative sleep. As an adult, your best deep sleep is usually between two a.m. and four a.m., in harmony with your body's circadian rhythm. When this rhythm gets disrupted, the quality of sleep changes, compromising the body's ability to restore itself.

To treat any form of sleep disturbance, you must first find its cause. Here are two common ones:

In a *deviated septum*, the piece of cartilage that separates the two halves of your nose gets pushed to one side of the nose or the other. If you have a deviated septum, you may feel chronic congestion in your nose, or one side of your nose may feel more blocked than the other. The only way to correct a deviated septum is to surgically fix it, so if you think you might have this problem, see an ear, nose, and throat (ENT) doctor who can realign the septum to the correct position and get you breathing better.

In *sleep apnea*, the soft part of the back of your throat and your tongue block the airway when you sleep. Sleep apnea can cause chronic snoring and periods during the night when you stop breathing for several seconds.

New home technologies like the Fitbit can measure if you have periods in the night where you are not breathing, and record how many times and for how long. Many people with sleep apnea feel tired when they wake, even if they felt like they slept well in the night. If you think you might have sleep apnea and do not have a home device to measure it, see a sleep specialist who can do an in-home or in-office sleep study that measures your breathing rate, the amount of oxygen in your blood, and whether you stop breathing in the night. If you find out you have sleep apnea, your doctor may prescribe a medical device called continuous positive airway pressure (CPAP), which is a mask you wear at night to help keep your airway open and stop sleep apnea. Alternatively, for those who cannot use a CPAP, you can have a dental mouthpiece made that repositions your jaw while you sleep to keep your airway open. Both work well in stopping sleep apnea and helping you get a more restful, deeper sleep.

Sleep Issues and Hormone Deficiencies

Hormone deficiencies such as low thyroid or abnormal adrenal function (or low estrogen or progesterone) can also affect sleep quality. If your thyroid is sluggish and underactive (hypothyroid), you may experience more fatigue during the day, insomnia, constipation, weight gain, cold hands and feet, dry skin, swelling under your eyes or ankles, hair loss, moodiness or depression, or an enlarged thyroid gland (called a goiter) in your neck. An overactive thyroid (hyperthyroid), on the other hand, can cause heart palpitations, diarrhea, sweating without exercising, weight loss, insomnia, tremors in your hands, hyperactivity, moodiness, anxiety, or bulging eyes. When your thyroid is underactive, you are more prone to sleep apnea, which interferes with getting a good night's sleep. But if your thyroid is overactive, the constant stimulation it causes prevents you from falling asleep and keeps you from getting deep, restful sleep.

With abnormal adrenal function, your cortisol levels are not in sync with your circadian rhythm. Cortisol should be at its highest levels somewhere between six a.m. and eight a.m. and at its lowest just before bedtime. However, if this pattern gets disrupted and your cortisol is being produced at the wrong times, you may have difficulty going to bed before midnight, wake in the middle of the night, or wake up too early. Many people with adrenal problems also feel like they have restless sleep and never sleep deeply.

Changes in estrogen and progesterone levels also have a big impact on women's sleep. This is why so many women start having sleep problems when they go through menopause, as their hormone levels naturally drop. Although this is common during menopause, younger women with Lyme disease often have irregular periods as well as sleep problems. Our brains have receptors for both estrogen and progesterone, so when these hormones start to decrease, you can feel mood changes, memory problems, anxiety, and sleep disturbances. But since women have so much more estrogen and progesterone than men do, they are much more likely to feel the changes in these hormones than men.

If you feel you might suffer from any of these hormone imbalances, see your doctor to find out if that explains why you haven't been sleeping well. A simple blood test can determine if your sleep issues are in part hormonal.

If the tests uncover any kind of hormonal imbalance, you must correct it. In some cases, nutrients or herbs can help do this. In more severe cases, hormone replacement may be the best option. A good naturopathic or functional medicine doctor can help you restore balance to your hormones in the safest, most natural way.

Nutrients and Supplements for Better Sleep

When it comes to formulas for better sleep, there is no magic potion that helps everybody. Prescription medications for sleep have many unwanted side effects. Although they may get you to sleep, they don't necessarily improve its quality. There have been numerous reports of people on prescription sleep medications waking in the night and getting in the car and driving somewhere or eating an entire loaf of bread with no recollection of having done so. Fortunately, certain nutrients and supplements can help you have deeper, more restorative sleep, but be patient with these interventions. Depending on how long you've had poor-quality sleep, it can take several weeks or months to get your body back on track.

Begin with the first supplement listed, and if that does not improve your sleep, then move on in turn to each of the following supplements for at least six weeks to see if it improves your sleep. If there has been no change at all in your sleep after six weeks, then it's time to try something different. Using single nutrients is easiest. But sometimes one nutrient isn't enough and you have to be a bit more aggressive. In that case it's fine to try combining nutrients. If you wake up in the morning feeling more tired, have lower energy during the day, or start to have fitful sleep, these can be signs that you are getting too much rest. You should either decrease the dose or cut one of the nutrients out. This list gives the recommended doses for each of the supplements, but if you are still struggling to find the right one, talk with your nutritionally oriented doctor.

Melatonin

If you have difficulty falling asleep, start with low doses of melatonin, a natural hormone that helps bring on sleep. Adults should start with 3 milligrams before bedtime and children with 1 milligram. Several studies have shown that melatonin supplements are safe for children and help them fall asleep faster.[2] Melatonin is safe and can even help control pain. If you take an immediate-release form of melatonin, it will get you to sleep but won't help you stay asleep. For this reason, use a continuous-release form, which releases melatonin in increments over the course of the night. Start with 5 milligrams, decreasing your dose if you feel groggy the next day.

GABA

Your brain chemistry consists of certain chemicals that stimulate the brain and others that quiet it down. A key molecule that helps your brain calm down is gamma-aminobutyric acid (GABA). Some people fall asleep more easily when they take GABA before bedtime. Interestingly, there is no research to suggest that GABA ever makes it to the brain, so we don't know why or how it works when taken as a supplement. Nonetheless, many people I've worked with report that they sleep better when they take GABA, and it is safe. Start with 750 milligrams at bedtime, increasing it up to 1,500 milligrams if needed. If you take too much GABA, it can make you feel groggy when you wake up, so if that happens, just decrease your dose.

Magnesium

Magnesium, one of the most-used nutrients in the body, is active in almost every metabolic pathway. It aids in energy metabolism, stress management, sleep, blood flow, gastrointestinal function, breathing, and heart rhythm. During stressful times, the body burns through a lot of magnesium, and the shortage can then amplify the effects of stress. This keeps the body in a constant state of fight or flight. Magnesium supplementation can help reduce the excitement in the brain and make it easier for the nervous system to calm down. Start with 100 milligrams of magnesium citrate twice a day. You can increase the amount, if tolerated, up to 250 milligrams twice a day. Too much magnesium will cause loose stools; if that happens, reduce the dose a little. Or try other forms of magnesium, such as magnesium taurate, magnesium threonate, or magnesium glycinate.

Passionflower

Many herbs can help induce sleep. One of my favorites, passionflower (*Passiflora incarnata*), helps with anxiety, stress, mood, and sleep. Native to North America, it grows throughout the Midwest of the United States. You can buy passionflower as a liquid tincture or in capsule form. At bedtime, take thirty drops of the liquid tincture or 700 milligrams of the capsules. Passionflower can also be useful for restlessness, including restless legs syndrome, which many people with Lyme experience in the evening.

Ashwagandha

Another herb that works well for people with Lyme disease who are "tired and wired" is ashwagandha (*Withania somnifera*), known as Indian ginseng. This ancient Indian plant has been used medicinally for thousands of years to treat fatigue, inflammation, pain, and stress. This is especially helpful for people who cannot sleep because they just cannot turn their brains off at night, even though they are physically exhausted. Ashwagandha is an adaptogen, which means it helps balance the effects of stress. Take 800 to 1,200 milligrams a day to reduce your stress hormones and allow your body to get into a more relaxed state before bed. For best results, take 400 to 600 milligrams at bedtime and the other half in the morning.

5-HTP

If your major problem is waking in the night, then 5-hydroxytryptophan (5-HTP) may help you to stay asleep. An amino acid, 5-HTP is a biological precursor to serotonin and melatonin, both of which improve sleep quality. Research shows that 5-HTP also helps people with depression and anxiety.[3] Like many people with Lyme, you may experience mood and emotional issues as well as sleep disturbances. If so, 5-HTP can help get your brain back in balance. Start with 100 milligrams of 5-HTP at bedtime. If your sleep has not improved, you can increase the dose every two weeks by 100 milligrams—up to 300 milligrams per night. If you wake up feeling groggy after taking 5-HTP or feel more tired in the morning, reduce the dose by 100 milligrams to the amount you were taking before you started feeling groggy.

Theanine

Green tea has many known health benefits. It contains a compound called theanine that calms anxiety and stress while helping you sleep.[4] It also helps improve mood and concentration.[5] Since theanine does not generally make people feel drowsy, you can take theanine during a workday or school day. It won't interfere with your daily activities. It also helps some people with Lyme get off their prescription medications for sleep or anxiety. However, do not stop your medications without first consulting your doctor. You can get serious withdrawal symptoms if you stop too rapidly. Take 200 milligrams at bedtime and another 200 milligrams during the day if needed for anxiety or stress. Please note that taking theanine is not the same as drinking green tea, which when taken before bedtime could interfere with your sleep. I recommend taking theanine as a nutritional supplement instead.

Valerian

Valerian root (*Valeriana officinalis*) is one of the most well-known natural sleep aids. It can help you fall asleep faster and stay asleep and does not typically leave you with a "sleep hangover" in the morning, like some prescription medications. Valerian may enhance the effect of GABA, although the research is not conclusive. To receive the full benefit of valerian, you may need to take it for as long as three weeks. Take 250 to 600 milligrams at bedtime. Some people get a paradoxical reaction to valerian—it actually makes them feel anxious and nervous. Stop taking it if this happens to you.

. . . .

Three Tips for Great Sleep

1. Go to bed at the same time every night. Your body has a biological clock that needs to be reset. Going to bed at a regular time will help get you back on a regular sleep pattern.
2. Avoid stimulants after dinner. Many people like a nice after-dinner cup of tea or coffee, but these contain caffeine. Because caffeine acts as a brain stimulant, it may often prevent you from being able to fall asleep. Instead choose caffeine-free herbal teas or hot water with lemon.
3. Try meditation. Several studies show that regular meditation can:
   - Relieve the effects of stress[6]
   - Reduce blood pressure and heart rate[7]
   - Reduce anxiety[8]
   - Promote better sleep[9]
   - Relieve pain[10]

Meditation takes some practice, but you'll find that it can help you relax your mind and get it ready for bed. As little as five or ten minutes at any time of day can be enough to get these healthy benefits. (You will find more about meditation toward the end of this chapter, in the section on stress management.)

. . . .

Reduce Your Exposure to Electronics

Some people are quite sensitive to electromagnetic waves. Electromagnetic waves, also known as electromagnetic frequencies (EMFs), are types of energy emitted from electronic devices such as cell phones, cordless phones, routers, and any electronic devices that can be connected without a cord. They also come from electrical outlets in the wall and high-tension wires in your neighborhood. In other words, they are all around almost all the time. Advances in computer and electrical technology have led to the ubiquity of wireless devices (such as smart meters to measure your home's electrical or gas use), which can have detrimental effects on some people.

According to the World Health Organization, there is little evidence showing a link between long-term EMF exposure and health risks.[11] However, that research was conducted in 1996. Newer research shows that chronic EMF exposure has been associated with certain types of cancer, Alzheimer's disease, male infertility, headaches, poor concentration, depression, sleep problems, and fatigue.[12] That's why some people attain better sleep when they reduce their exposure to electromagnetic radiation at night. In other words, turn off your smartphone, iPad, and laptop. Unplug the Wi-Fi altogether. Reducing your exposure to Wi-Fi may help you enjoy a more restful sleep.

In fact, it's best to turn your electronics off two hours before bedtime. Why? The new high-resolution screens emit a blue light that, when used at night, tricks the brain into thinking it's daytime. Turning off electronic screens well in advance of your bedtime will make it easier for you to fall asleep. It will give your brain a chance to adjust to the fact that it is actually nighttime and not the eternal present of the Internet. Most smartphones and tablets have a feature you can turn on to minimize blue light at night. Or you can purchase glasses from several online stores, such as Amazon, that filter out blue light. Reading a good book before bedtime can do wonders to help take your mind off the day, without overstimulating your brain the way that looking at a high-resolution multimedia screen does.

If Nothing Works

If you've tried all these suggestions and find that you still have difficulty sleeping, see a sleep specialist to help determine the cause of your poor sleep. As I've mentioned earlier, there may be anatomical causes, such as a deviated septum, or other physiological problems, such as sleep apnea. A sleep specialist will help you figure out why you don't sleep well and can offer additional forms of treatment. Although it's usually advisable to avoid pharmaceuticals, chronic insomnia and poor sleep are much harder on your body than most sleep medications. If you do need a prescription, talk with your doctor about starting with the lowest dose to help minimize any potential side effects.

Exercise Your Way Back to a Stronger You

Prior to contracting Lyme disease, I was an athletic person who always participated in competitive sports. But after getting infected with Lyme, I experienced such debilitating fatigue that the mere thought of doing anything physically active was exhausting. Suddenly I had no strength or endurance. Even the smallest amount of activity would tire me out. Fortunately, as I started to recover, I was able to do a little more. Short walks and house chores seemed doable again. Once my stamina increased, I was able to do physical activity for longer periods. Eventually I began training in karate, finally receiving my black belt almost six years after my tick bite. Had you asked me early in my Lyme journey if I believed that the day would come when that was possible, I would have said you were crazy. But as I got better control over my Lyme, exercise became a regular part of my life and played an essential role in my healing.

I know that many of you have felt or feel the same way. The mental and physical effects of Lyme disease make it hard to sustain a regular exercise routine. Some people lack the motivation to exercise. Others lack the physical strength. Whatever your obstacle, it is important to understand how exercise helps you overcome Lyme disease. Once you start moving your body, blood flow increases, which means more oxygen and nutrients get delivered to the areas that need them most. Increased blood flow and nutrients help your body repair and restore damaged cells. Lyme disease tends to make your blood thick.[13] That's why regular exercise helps your blood move more easily. Other benefits are improving mood and sleep, as well as boosting your immune system.[14]

The key is to start gently. Because Lyme often causes issues with so many body systems at one time, any type of vigorous aerobic exercise can backfire, making you feel much worse. Always check in with yourself and assess honestly how you are feeling. Try not to overextend yourself as you continue to improve and feel better. Many people with Lyme start to feel better, then proceed to work out too hard. Often they end up in bed for weeks with terrible fatigue, joint pain, muscle aches, or headaches. Pushing your body beyond its capacities only works against you, so be patient. Listen to those cues that tell you you've done too much, and rest.

Walking

The best way to start your exercise program is to simply walk. You may find that you can walk only short distances or for a few minutes. That's okay. Don't try to climb hills or steep streets. Try to find a level surface, so you don't overexert yourself. If your neighborhood is hilly, seek out a local school with an outdoor track or go to a mall for indoor walking. If you have difficulties with balance, use a cane for support or walk with a friend who can help you if you feel unbalanced. Even a few laps around your home can help. The main thing is to move your body. Any movement is better than none at all.

Yoga

Yoga is a wonderful form of gentle exercise. Practiced for more than two thousand years by millions of people worldwide, it involves performing a series of physical postures that can be easily modified for each individual, so it's ideal for any fitness level. Health benefits include increased strength, flexibility, and balance; deeper breathing; and more energy. Yoga decreases stress and weight. It integrates the mind and the body to produce better physical and mental health. With so many different styles of yoga, it is relatively easy to find one that best suits your exercise tolerance. Most people with Lyme disease can do beginner-level yoga poses. Various types, or schools, of yoga (such as hatha, Iyengar, and others) entail holding certain specific postures while standing, seated, or lying down. Beginner-level yoga moves at a slower pace than more advanced forms in order to help you learn the poses and build strength and flexibility. More advanced forms of yoga, such as Bikram or "hot" yoga, or anything fast-paced, aerobic, or strenuous, is best avoided by people with Lyme disease.

Another option for people with Lyme disease is restorative yoga, a gentler, slower-paced style. Restorative yoga (as it sounds) is designed to help you relax, restore energy, and get all the benefits of yoga even if you are weak, injured, or out of shape. You may experience more immediate calming and meditative effects than when you do other more physically demanding types of yoga. In a restorative yoga class, you may do only five or six poses, supported by props that take some of the physical stress off your body so you can hold the poses longer. Props may include chairs, blankets, pillows, blocks, straps, balls, or towels, allowing you to feel supported and comfortable in each position. Each pose may be held for about five minutes and involves light twists, seated forward bending, or gentle back bends. You may need to make small adjustments in your props to feel comfortable. The placement of your body is important. Modifying the pose by as little as half an inch can make the difference between feeling comfortable and having pain. Yoga may take a little practice to find out what works best for you, but stick with it and you'll find it gets easier the longer you do it. Many Iyengar yoga teachers also offer restorative yoga classes.

Swimming

If you find it difficult to walk or your balance is poor, swimming may be a better way to get your body going. Being in salt water can be very healing. With my own bout of Lyme, I found that after swimming in a saltwater pool, the neuropathy I had experienced decreased. This method of getting your exercise is more expensive, since you have to find a pool in your area and you will probably have to pay for a membership, but if that is an option for you, it can be a very good way to get moving. Swimming builds muscle and improves endurance. You can also modify your swimming routine to be as easy or difficult as you feel you can handle. Freestyle, backstroke, and sidestroke can all be done at a slow pace, so you don't get fatigued too easily. Using a kickboard to help keep your head above water is a great way to swim without having to hold your breath and may be easier for you as you start. Many individuals with Lyme are chemically sensitive, so if you do have a choice, it's a good idea to avoid chlorinated pools in favor of saltwater pools.

Tai Chi and Qi Gong

Tai chi was originally developed as a Chinese martial art but has evolved into an easygoing series of gentle, standing movements, which you learn to coordinate with deep breathing. Each movement flows into the next in a slow, rhythmic manner. While it may sound very similar to yoga, the poses are quite different. Since the joints are never fully extended, tai chi requires much less strength than yoga and is less stressful on the joints and muscles. It is so gentle, it can even be done by the elderly. In China, people in their late eighties and nineties can be seen doing it every morning in public parks. Because it emphasizes relaxation as part of the exercise, tai chi has been described as "meditation in motion."

A variation on tai chi called qi gong also involves slow, gentle movements but uses more static poses. The same poses are repeated multiple times or held longer. Both of these ancient Chinese practices can help improve stamina and flexibility while helping you ease your stress and relax your mind. Classes are offered in most cities.

Start any exercise program slowly and increase the intensity or duration as you feel your body can handle it. Be mindful of how you feel during and after exercising, so you can modify your program the next time. If you are exhausted for days after exercising, it was too much and you need to decrease the intensity or length of your workout. You'll be surprised how quickly your strength and energy increase once you get into a regular routine. Consistency is the key. Try to work up to exercising three to five days per week if tolerated. But remember, any movement is helpful. Small steps can lead to big changes.

Stress Management: Finding Peace in Your Chaos

Sleep and exercise have multiple benefits, among them their ability to reduce stress levels. But there are also several tools, like meditation and biofeedback, that you can learn to use to reduce your stress response directly. They can also be immensely helpful in some cases to relieve the stress of your illness—and the stress it may also be causing your network of family and friends. Many people with Lyme benefit from going to a support group or professional therapist to cope with the stress of having Lyme.

Meditation

Years of research have proven that meditation can help relieve much of the tension that you carry during your day. It not only helps you get better sleep but also helps reduce your stress hormones. If you have a hard time sitting quietly by yourself, you might be helped by guided meditation, where you listen to someone else's voice as they take you through a series of mental images and thoughts to help calm your brain. With another voice to focus on, you are less likely to daydream or have your mind wander off. Bernie Siegel, MD, a former cancer surgeon, has created a series of guided meditation programs that have helped many people to relax and de-stress.

Biofeedback

Biofeedback has also helped many individuals with Lyme disease learn how to relieve stress by developing more conscious control over their bodies in order to move into a relaxed state. In biofeedback, you are trained to improve your health by measuring different signals from your body and then learning how to change those signals with your mind. For example, if you have a tight muscle, the biofeedback device may detect that it is tight, and then you can learn how to focus on getting that muscle to relax. Many biofeedback devices hook electrodes up to different parts of the body to measure heart rate, skin temperature, and other bodily functions, but other ways exist to train your brain that don't involve being connected to a piece of equipment. Many practitioners provide biofeedback services, but there are also some good online or smartphone applications that can be used without having to see a professional. The success of biofeedback is related to the frequency of sessions: you need to do it at least two to three times per week at the start. As with most therapies, the more you do it, the better results you get.

Relationships

If the stress of Lyme disease is taking a toll on your relationships, get help outside your circle of family and friends. Many cities around the world have Lyme support groups, where you can meet with others who share similar life circumstances, fears, and feelings. Having a safe place to talk with others about what goes on in your mind, or just a place to get emotional support, can be invaluable. Support groups can also provide a place to share treatment ideas and experiences with other practitioners or therapies. Such groups give you the opportunity to freely express yourself with others who do not judge you for what you think or feel. Those with Lyme disease share a common bond. Many of you have been in that dark place wondering whether you'll ever feel better. Support groups can give you the comfort and emotional strength to keep working on your health and inspire you to try new things. Find a local Lyme support group that meets regularly. If you do not have a local group, look for online Lyme support groups, so you can connect with others no matter where you are in the world. Please visit lymedis ease.org or lymediseasesupportnetwork.org to get online support. You can also visit my website at dariningelsnd.com and click the link for online support.

If you don't feel comfortable in group settings, it can be valuable to meet with a psychotherapist or counselor. Some people prefer the one-on-one interaction that feels more personal to them. I worked with a wonderful local therapist for over a year and found the sessions extremely helpful. It was such a relief to have an impartial person to share my concerns and fears and then have them reframed for me from a different perspective. For example, when I went through the "why me?" phase, she was able to reframe that question as an opportunity to make changes in my own life to have better health. Having that go-to person when you're feeling down in the dumps can help lift your spirits and shed new light on your life. It may seem unnatural to share your innermost thoughts and secrets with a complete stranger, but these professionals are trained to help you find ways to let go of the things that bother you or hold you back from getting well. As with any relationship, sometimes you click with a therapist and sometimes you don't. There's nothing wrong with meeting a few people to see who the best fit is for you. With the right person, you can relieve stress while getting guidance to better manage your emotional health.

Take Control of What You Can

There are so many aspects of Lyme disease that are beyond your control. No one chose to get infected and suffer the consequences of a tick bite. But understand that you have the ability to make changes in your life that can help you start to feel well again. Making lifestyle changes can be difficult. Breaking old bad habits and instituting a new plan of action in your life can take time. Every step you take to making healthier lifestyle choices is a step toward recovery. Remember, each of the factors discussed in this chapter plays some role in the way that you feel and the way that you heal. Although you may not feel that any one thing is making much of a difference, the additive effect of making all of these changes can produce big outcomes.

Starting new, healthy habits can be challenging, so keep in mind that not all changes will happen immediately. Some changes will come more easily than others—for example, getting the mold out of your house is a big project. But other changes are fully within your power to begin now. Don't get discouraged. And don't be afraid to ask for help, whether it's from your health-care provider, your family, or your friends. Please see the Resources section (page 325) for extra support.

Part Three

· ·

Treating Chronic Lyme

In Part Three, we will concentrate on additional treatment for the most chronic and persistent cases of Lyme disease—as well as tips for going through another round of the program to upgrade your results. With the solid foundations and improvements already received from following the Five-Stage Immune-Boosting Plan, many people will have experienced a solid recovery. Still, if you still have a way to go, remember that your immune system may have taken a real battering from many rounds of antibiotics. You may therefore need to repeat the program to get additional results. You may also need to consider going for some advanced therapies available from Lyme-literate practitioners. In the two chapters of Part Three, I will cover both of these options.

Chapter 8 offers advanced protocols for treating chronic Lyme. Here I introduce three powerhouse therapies for which you will need the guidance of a health-care professional. If you are nearly all the way to recovery, you might skip this chapter and move directly to Chapter 9, which offers guidance for recycling through the Immune-Boosting Plan to enhance your recovery.

Advanced Protocols

The Five-Stage Immune-Boosting Plan I've offered in Part Two can be safely followed by anyone seeking to overcome Lyme disease. The Immune-Boosting Diet may also help in strengthening the immune system to reduce vulnerability to getting Lyme disease.

Throughout the book, I've offered my most successful strategies to strengthen your immune system and reduce the burden of the Lyme organism in your body. The goal of this program is to feed your cells nutritionally and give your immune system every opportunity to do what nature intends. As you move through different parts of the program, you may experience some relief. You may also find that certain symptoms are stubborn and don't go away as quickly or easily as others. The most challenging symptoms for many people who have Lyme are persistent fatigue and neuropathy. This chapter will present great approaches to overcome these obstacles.

The purpose of this book is to empower you to take control of your own health, give you tools to overcome Lyme disease, and help you get well. While you can follow many of these advanced protocols on your own, in some cases—which I will note—you will need to consult a health-care provider who is familiar with the treatments presented in this chapter or can offer other treatments that require medical supervision. The Resources section (page 325) will help you locate a practitioner knowledgeable in these approaches.

As you've learned throughout this book, in early acute Lyme disease, antibiotic therapy may succeed in killing the spirochetes before your immune system responds. In chronic Lyme disease, the activation of your immune system itself is causing the symptoms, leading to an autoimmune disorder. That is why the core of my prescription is to rebalance your immune system and modulate its overreactive attack on your own organs and tissues. Because the shape-shifting Lyme bug makes it nearly impossible to kill all forms of Lyme infection once and for all, this is the most sensible and effective way to regain your health.

In this chapter, I'm going to introduce you to some advanced tools available for balancing and calming your immune system. They are highly effective in clinical practice. I will cover various forms of immunotherapy that can help you get over your allergies and sensitivities and put your immune system back in good working order. This chapter will also discuss some novel ways to take the burden off your immune system and change the way it reacts to triggers.

Yet because of conventional medicine's narrow focus on killing bugs, these methods are not widely known or used. As you have discovered from following the protocols in Chapter 5, killing bugs is important—but it's not always enough. These recommendations can be added to your Lyme protocol to help you overcome the following specific symptoms if the earlier recommendations in this book have not fully resolved them.

Because chronic fatigue is the most common symptom pattern that accompanies Lyme disease, let's begin with that.

How to Overcome Chronic Fatigue

Chronic fatigue disrupts the daily lives of almost all people with Lyme disease. It interferes with their ability to bathe, cook, shop, and clean. Although there are many possible explanations for the fatigue, in many people it is related to any or all of the following:

- Underactive thyroid[1]
- Poor sleep patterns[2]
- Poor or inadequate nutrition[3]
- Depression[4]
- Mitochondrial dysfunction[5]

In previous chapters of this book, you read about the first four of these factors. The fifth, mitochondrial dysfunction, is far less well known. The inside of our cells contain many microscopic parts, all of which have a specific function in making the cell work. The mitochondria are one of those cell parts responsible for making energy. They produce a key molecule, adenosine 5′-triphosphate (ATP), which supplies energy to your cells. Without enough ATP, your cells and organs don't function well and start to get tired. When mitochondria, which are found in almost every cell in your body, are damaged or don't function properly, every tissue or organ they supply with energy suffers. Defects in mitochondria have been associated with almost every chronic illness, including autism, Parkinson's disease, multiple sclerosis, Lou Gehrig's disease (ALS), diabetes, fibromyalgia, chronic fatigue syndrome, and heart disease.[6]

Although some people are born with genetic mitochondrial diseases, like Leigh syndrome, carnitine deficiency, or coenzyme Q10 deficiency, such illnesses are typically identified early in life. These are not the types of mitochondrial illness seen with Lyme disease.

Studies have shown that Lyme disease can reduce the number of, as well as damage, your mitochondria.[7] This results in reduced ATP production—and therefore a lack of energy. The good news is that several nutrients can repair your mitochondria and support their function. This process is not quick and can take weeks or months, but if you take these nutrients consistently, you will get the best and fastest results. Some of them can interfere with certain medications, so it's best to get advice from a naturopathic physician or functional medicine practitioner who knows about drug-nutrient interactions. I've listed these supplements in the order I recommend trying them.

Coenzyme Q10 (CoQ10)

CoQ10 is a nutrient you need to make ATP, the body's main form of energy storage. It is naturally found in many foods but only in small quantities. Food sources of CoQ10 include organ meats such as liver, kidney, and heart; poultry; fish; nuts; eggs; and some fruits and vegetables. CoQ10 is a potent antioxidant, which protects against heart disease and cancer, but research shows that it is also an important nutrient for the immune system. Other studies have shown that CoQ10 helps treat the following:

- Heart disease[8]
- High blood pressure[9]
- Hyperthyroidism[10]
- Migraine headaches[11]
- Alzheimer's disease[12]
- Parkinson's disease[13]

- AIDS[14]
- Hearing loss[15]
- Ringing in the ears[16]

People who take certain medications must also be cautious, as some can lead to depletion of CoQ10. Perhaps the most well-studied drug-nutrient interaction is between statin drugs and CoQ10. Numerous studies have shown that statin medications lower CoQ10 levels.[17] That may be why people who take these drugs get muscle pain and heart problems. So if you take a statin drug for high cholesterol, it would be wise to supplement with CoQ10. Other medications known to interfere with CoQ10 include the following:

- Beta blockers—used to treat high blood pressure
- Warfarin—used as a blood thinner for heart disease or blood clots
- Doxorubicin—used as part of many chemotherapy protocols for cancer
- Zidovudine—used to treat HIV/AIDS
- Gentamycin—used to treat certain infections
- Nucleoside reverse transcriptase inhibitors (NRTIs)—used to treat HIV/AIDS

CoQ10 is a fat-soluble nutrient, which means you need to have a little fat in your diet when you take this as a nutritional supplement. There are several forms of CoQ10, but you will mostly find it in granular form (ubiquinone) or oil-based (ubiquinol). Some companies argue that the oil-based form is better absorbed, but studies are inconclusive. Nevertheless, I have seen good results using this form of CoQ10.

To get your energy back, start with 100 milligrams of CoQ10 in the morning with breakfast and another 100 milligrams with lunch. You can increase the dose as needed, up to 600 milligrams twice a day. CoQ10 is well tolerated and may cause mild gastrointestinal side effects at higher doses. Once you start to feel that your energy is better, stay with that dose. Don't take CoQ10 after dinner—it can stimulate energy metabolism and interfere with your sleep. If you take it with breakfast and lunch, you are less likely to have any adverse sleep changes from it. If you find your sleep pattern does change for the worse, then decrease the dose by 100 milligrams until you are sleeping well again.

Carnitine

Carnitine is another nutrient that supports your mitochondria and can give you more energy. About 98 percent of all the carnitine in your body is found in your muscles and heart. It transports fatty acids into the mitochondria, which allows them to convert those fatty acids into energy. Like CoQ10, carnitine can enhance immune function and is active in detoxification. Carnitine deficiency is common and can be caused by too little of it in the diet, poor absorption in the gut, chronic infections, a ketogenic diet (a high-fat, low-carb diet), liver disease, and use of certain medications. Signs of carnitine deficiency include fatigue, muscle weakness, low blood sugar, and a buildup of fat in your organs—commonly in your liver.

A recent study found that people with Lyme disease who had neurological symptoms, such as memory problems, mood changes, poor balance, and neuropathy, had lower blood levels of carnitine compared with people who were free of Lyme disease and healthy.[18] Lower levels were also seen in people with post-Lyme syndrome. Those with severe Lyme had lower levels than those with acute Lyme. We don't know why Lyme decreases blood carnitine levels, but this has been observed with other chronic infections as well.

About 75 percent of all carnitine comes from the diet. Only 25 percent is made directly in the body, so to regain your strength and stamina, make sure you get enough carnitine. Carnitine is found almost exclusively in animal foods, particularly beef, pork, fish, chicken, and milk products. Unfortunately, most of these foods are acidic, which is why it's usually preferable to get carnitine through supplementation. Some medications can deplete the body of carnitine, including valproic acid, which is used to treat seizures, and some chemotherapy medications.

Carnitine can be found in two forms, L-carnitine and acetyl-L-carnitine. L-carnitine is the biologically active form, but acetyl-L-carnitine seems to penetrate the brain better than L-carnitine. Studies in rats show that acetyl-L-carnitine is a better antioxidant than L-carnitine, so acetyl-L-carnitine may provide other health benefits beyond just enhancing your energy.[19] Start with 1,000 milligrams of acetyl-L-carnitine per day in the morning. Add another 1,000 milligrams at lunch if you do not feel any change in your energy after two weeks. It is best to take it in divided doses. Carnitine is well tolerated, but at high doses it can cause nausea or diarrhea. Some people report that they develop an unpleasant body odor that smells fishy. If any of these symptoms happen to you, the side effects should resolve if you cut your dose back by 500 milligrams.

WESLEY'S STORY

Wes was diagnosed with autism when he was eighteen months old. Over the years, he saw multiple doctors who worked with his diet, supplements, and other medications to enable him to function better. His parents always described him as a "floppy" kid.

He found it hard to climb, run, and jump like other kids. His parents told me that Wes would nap whenever he was given the chance, which was an issue when he was in his therapy sessions, as he was unable to stay focused and do what was asked of him. He also had difficulties with language. At age six, he spoke only a handful of words. Although he had numerous tests done over the years, he had never been tested for Lyme disease. After his Lyme test came back positive, Wes began to follow the Immune-Boosting Diet and take an herbal protocol for the infection.

I next started Wes on 100 milligrams of CoQ10, 100 milligrams of magnesium, 50 milligrams of vitamin B6, 500 milligrams of acetyl-L-carnitine, and 5 milligrams of NADH. His parents noticed that his energy started to improve over the next four weeks. They also noticed that he tried to use new words and imitated his sister more. His therapists all commented on how much better he did in his sessions and how he reached his goals much faster. I kept Wes on this cocktail of nutrients for several months, and we watched his energy, cognition, and language improve. As his mitochondria were reactivated, his whole body began to work well again.

Wes is now twelve years old. He continues to learn new skills. He has not had any issues with his energy. He is in a mainstream school with an aide and keeps up with other kids in his classroom. He is a good example of what can happen when you just put a little gas in an empty tank.

Alpha-Lipoic Acid

Alpha-lipoic acid (ALA) is a cofactor for enzymes that work to maximize your mitochondria's energy output. Cofactors are helper molecules needed for certain reactions. ALA is also an antioxidant. It works in conjunction with other antioxidants such as vitamin C, vitamin E, and glutathione to protect cells against damage. Often, it is given to people who have excess amounts of iron or copper in their bodies, in order to reduce the blood levels of those metals to safe amounts. It has been used to treat hepatitis, burning-mouth syndrome, and vitiligo. There is also good research that ALA can reduce blood sugar and prevent neuropathy in diabetics.[20]

Although there is no specific research on the use of ALA for Lyme disease or chronic fatigue, in my experience it improves energy in individuals with Lyme who are always tired. It is generally well tolerated with rare side effects. A small number of people may develop gastrointestinal distress or low blood sugar after they take ALA and have to decrease their dose or stop. People who are deficient in vitamin B1 (thiamine) may be more at risk of developing side effects, so taking a vitamin supplement containing vitamin B1 before you take ALA may be a good idea. Take 200 to 600 milligrams a day in divided doses. You can take higher doses, but because of the potential effects on blood sugar, only do so under the supervision of your health-care provider.

Vitamin B6 and Magnesium: The One-Two Punch for More Energy

If you look at a metabolic map, a chart that shows how all of the chemicals in your body interact with one another, you will see that vitamin B6 (pyridoxine) and magnesium are cofactors for almost every metabolic pathway that produces energy.

It's common to have deficiencies in both of these nutrients, so if you don't get enough of them in your diet, it will be more difficult to make the right molecules to increase your energy levels. Your body uses both of these nutrients to make thyroid hormone, dopamine, and adrenaline, all of which are necessary for good energy.

Good research shows that vitamin B6 boosts energy.[21] When taken with magnesium, vitamin B6 helps magnesium get inside the cells. Once inside the cell, magnesium is able to turn on ATP and produce more energy. The capacity of these supplements to turn on mitochondria has also been seen in children with autism. Bernie Rimland, PhD, studied the effects of vitamin B6 and magnesium in autistic children back in the 1960s.[22] He found that most of the children improved their language, eye contact, and awareness. They also had fewer tantrums and engaged in less self-injurious behavior. Years later, it's now better known that many children with autism have mitochondrial issues, the likely reason that this nutrient combination improved their mitochondrial function.[23] I too have worked with autistic children and can confirm that the combination of these two nutrients works well.

You can find vitamin B6 in the forms of both pyridoxine and pyridoxal-5-phosphate (P5P). Although P5P is the active form of vitamin B6, at least one study suggests pyridoxine is better absorbed.[24] In my experience, however, they both seem to work equally for most people. Start with 100 milligrams of vitamin B6 in the morning with breakfast. You can take higher doses, but B6 does have the potential to be toxic at high doses (usually more than 400 milligrams a day). If you take too much you may experience numbness and tingling in the arms and legs. Magnesium comes in many bound forms. Use either magnesium citrate or magnesium glycinate. These work well and are well tolerated. Start with 100 milligrams twice a day. Too much magnesium can cause loose stool or diarrhea, so decrease the dose, if needed. If you take magnesium in divided doses instead of all at once, this is less likely to happen.

NADH

Nicotinamide adenine dinucleotide (NADH) is another powerhouse that can increase energy in people with chronic fatigue syndrome. Many people with chronic fatigue have undiagnosed Lyme disease or co-infections. Not only will NADH improve your energy, it may also support cognitive function and memory.

Take 10 milligrams a day of NADH in the morning. Studies have found no additional benefit at higher doses, since it seems to get broken down in the intestines more readily before it is able to get absorbed across the gut wall. Side effects are minor, but some people report changes in their appetite, feel overstimulated, or have an unpleasant taste in their mouth on initially taking NADH supplements.

How to Overcome Neuropathy

Lyme disease can cause a type of *peripheral neuropathy*, a condition in which the electrical signals transmitted between nerves in the body and the brain or spinal cord get disrupted. This leads to various neurological symptoms, including numbness, tingling, pain, or a burning sensation in the skin, hands, or feet. Neuropathy is a hallmark of a number of illnesses, including multiple sclerosis, diabetes, alcoholism, Guillain-Barré syndrome, some cancers, lupus, and rheumatoid arthritis. It is also a side effect of certain drugs used to treat cancer or HIV. Many people who have Lyme disease, whether acute or chronic, experience neuropathy at some point in their illness. Neuropathy is also one of the most frustrating symptoms for individuals with Lyme, as it impairs the ability to walk, exercise, or hold on to things. It also affects your sensation of hot, cold, and pressure. The constant burning pain can disrupt your sleep and quality of life.

During my own Lyme journey, all of my symptoms disappeared completely before the neuropathy did. This occurs often in people with Lyme. It isn't clear why this particular symptom is more difficult to treat. Lyme disease affects the small nerve fibers in the body, which is why people experience vision problems, ringing in the ears, heart palpitations, and loss of balance. Depending on which nerves are involved, the symptoms of neuropathy can change. If your neuropathy has not improved by following the first part of the program, try these other interventions.

Phosphatidylcholine

Phosphatidylcholine (PC) is a specific fat molecule integral to almost every cell in your body, especially your brain and nerves. It makes up a large part of the outer part of the cell membrane. PC is also a precursor to one of your neurotransmitters, acetylcholine, which is necessary for normal nerve transmission. If something starts to break down this fatty molecule in the nerves, nerve conduction can be compromised, which can lead to symptoms of neuropathy. PC has been used to treat many conditions, including hepatitis C, ulcerative colitis, and some psychiatric disorders, such as bipolar disorder and Alzheimer's disease.[25]

Intake of this nutrient often helps neuropathy in individuals who have Lyme. PC can be taken as an oral supplement or administered intravenously. Start with 1,000 milligrams twice a day with food. Higher doses are appropriate in severe cases of neuropathy, but this should be done only under the guidance of your health-care provider. If you take any medications for Alzheimer's disease or glaucoma, be careful taking PC, as it may reduce the effectiveness of your medication.

If you are working with a nutritionally oriented physician who is knowledgeable about intravenous nutritional therapy, there is another option. PC can be administered intravenously, bypassing the gut and liver and therefore entering your cells more readily. This can be a powerhouse treatment for neuropathic symptoms, and many people with Lyme disease have benefited from it. Both the oral and IV PC are safe, so you can use either route. But be patient with this therapy. It may take six to eight weeks to see big improvements.

Glutathione

Glutathione is a three-amino-acid molecule that is one of the body's greatest antioxidants and liver detoxifiers. It supports your liver in the elimination of various toxins from your organs and cells. Most people with Lyme either are deficient in glutathione or have a genetic defect in glutathione metabolism that alters the way the body uses this molecule. Optimizing your glutathione levels gives your body every chance to detoxify, support your immune system, and repair damaged cells. Glutathione also works in conjunction with vitamin C in that they recycle each other in the cells.

Something called *reduced glutathione* works best. If glutathione gets oxidized, it becomes inactive and does nothing useful for you. Several companies have found ways to keep glutathione in its reduced (nonoxidized) state, to better deliver the health benefits. Tim Guilford, MD, of Los Altos, California, has developed a *liposomal glutathione*, a liquid form of glutathione packaged in small fatty molecules that allows for better absorption across the gut wall. It is absorbed almost as well in this form as it is intravenously. Glutathione has a sulfur-based amino acid in it called cysteine, which gives it a slight egg odor and taste. Take 1 milliliter one to two times a day mixed in a little juice. Once the bottle is opened, keep the bottle in the refrigerator so it won't oxidize and spoil.

If you cannot tolerate the smell or taste of liposomal glutathione, use S-acetyl-glutathione, an encapsulated form. Take 200 milligrams two to three times per day. Glutathione can also be administered intravenously or inhaled. Either method increases glutathione levels effectively. Again, if you are working with a nutritionally oriented physician, there is an additional option: getting glutathione injections. It can also be combined with PC. Taking these two nutrients together is even more effective than taking either on its own. No matter how you take it, glutathione stimulates detoxification. As a result, it may make you feel nauseated. If so, decrease the dose, and your symptoms will not recur the next time you take it. When, over time, you better tolerate it, you can then slowly increase the dose.

Vitamin B12

Most people with Lyme are deficient in vitamin B12, for reasons that are not clear—no research shows why Lyme might deplete the body of B12. Vitamin B12 does many things, and one of its roles is to protect the outer layer of our nerves, called the myelin sheath. The myelin allows the nerves to send signals from the brain to the rest of the body uninterrupted. It is similar to the plastic coating on electrical wires that allows the electricity to flow easily. If the plastic covering breaks, electricity does not flow downstream, and there is less power at the end of the wire. When the worn-out nerves don't work as well as they should, this can cause neuropathy. The wearing down of the myelin sheath also causes multiple sclerosis (MS), a reason that many people with Lyme are misdiagnosed with MS.

Vitamin B12, also known as cobalamin, is found almost exclusively in red meat, with much smaller amounts in eggs, dairy products, fish, and some poultry. Since on the Immune-Boosting Diet you will forgo most of the high-vitamin B12 foods because of their acidity, take vitamin B12 as a supplement. There are several forms of vitamin B12, including methylcobalamin, hydroxocobalamin, and cyanocobalamin. Methylcobalamin is the active form of vitamin B12 and the one most used. If you have done any genetic tests and know you have difficulties with methylation, then you may do better with hydroxocobalamin. Avoid cyanocobalamin, since it has a cyanide molecule attached to the vitamin B12 and may not be the safest form. Start with 1,000 micrograms per day of vitamin B12 taken under the tongue (sublingual). The absorption of vitamin B12 seems to be better when taken sublingually.

In addition to daily oral vitamin B12, some individuals benefit from weekly B12 injections. For some reason, giving the vitamin B12 directly in the muscle (intramuscular, or IM) has a better effect on neuropathy than just taking it by mouth. Vitamin B12 does not get stored in the body, so there is no toxicity when it's given this way. Talk with your doctor about whether using IM vitamin B12 is right for you. If so, take 1,000 micrograms intramuscularly two to three times per week when the neuropathy is severe. You are unlikely to experience any adverse side effect at this dose. It can take up to six weeks to see the full benefits, so do the injections for at least that long.

PEMF

Pulsed electromagnetic frequency (PEMF) therapy delivers low-level electromagnetic signals. Each cell in the body emits a very low-level frequency, which allows cells to communicate with each other. These low-level electromagnetic signals are important for good health. Other types of electromagnetic signals may be unhealthy for us. As I discussed in Chapter 7, in modern life, most people are regularly exposed to Wi-Fi, cell phones, and laptop computers. These devices emit EMFs that are vastly different from the human body's. As a result, some research shows that exposure to that type of EMF may disrupt normal organ function.[26] However, PEMF generates low-level frequencies that stimulate blood flow and tissue repair.[27] These frequencies resonate with our organs and cells to repair and restore their function.

For many years, European doctors have used PEMF to help heal broken bones.[28] More recently, PEMF has come into use in the United States for pain, stress, anxiety, and depression.[29] Although these devices do emit an electromagnetic field, don't confuse them with magnetic resonance imaging (MRI) or transcutaneous electrical nerve stimulation (TENS), which are used for different medical purposes.

Two categories of PEMF devices are sold in the United States, some for professional use and others for home use. The devices for home use have more limited capabilities. Nevertheless, if you don't have access to a practitioner with professional equipment, the consumer models do deliver results. All PEMF devices work in a similar way and are safe and effective. The length of treatment sessions can vary from a few minutes to more than an hour. The Lyme protocol I offer in my clinic runs about seventy-five minutes. I recommend that either on your own, or with a practitioner, you do PEMF treatments twice a week for six weeks. In the Resources section (page 325), I offer links to both practitioners and consumer devices.

MARINA'S STORY

Marina was referred to our practice from a local colleague who treated her Lyme disease for several months. She had been on antibiotics as well as a strict diet, with many nutritional supplements. Despite her treatment, Marina was unable to walk more than a few feet and used a wheelchair. She had started to lose hope and had already lost a large part of her life because of her illness.

When she came in, we decided to have her try PEMF therapy and low-dose immunotherapy. We wheeled her back to our treatment room and eased her onto the table to get set up with the PEMF treatment. She had a difficult time standing, because of muscle weakness along with neuropathy in her legs. We finally got her situated and hooked up for her session. We did the Lyme-specific protocol and added another protocol for stress.

After her treatment ended, she pulled her legs over the edge of the table and stood on her own. She then walked out of the room and down the hall. Her husband followed her with the wheelchair, but she insisted she did not need it. Marina said it was the first time in more than a year that she felt strong enough to walk on her own. Although she walked very slowly, she was able to walk out to the car. She called a few days later to tell us that she was still getting stronger and was not using the wheelchair at home. Marina's experience reveals that PEMF can produce a significant impact, even after one session. Although this dramatic effect is unusual, most people do feel better after each treatment.

IVIG

Intravenous immunoglobulin (IVIG) is a therapy that is used to treat various immune, autoimmune, and infectious diseases. It consists of highly concentrated amounts of antibodies that come from multiple blood donors, making it rich with mostly immunoglobulin G (95 percent) and small amounts of immunoglobulin M and immunoglobulin A (see page 242). Severe immune deficiency, some autoimmune diseases, and multiple sclerosis can also be addressed with this treatment. Given intravenously, the antibodies confer a higher boost of immunity than your body can create on its own. I have worked with several people over the years whose neuropathy really improved after IVIG when other therapies failed.

Unfortunately, there are several downsides to IVIG. Most insurance companies will not pay for the treatment unless you have a severe immune disorder. For individuals with Guillain-Barré syndrome, common variable immunodeficiency, Kawasaki's disease, certain types of cancer or leukemia, or idiopathic thrombocytopenic purpura (ITP), IVIG is usually covered. However, many people with Lyme do not fit those criteria. Costing up to $10,000 per treatment, the therapy is obviously very expensive. It can take up to six treatments to see improvement. The other downside is that IVIG is made from the blood of many donors and, like any blood product, carries its own risk of blood-borne disease. The blood supply is screened for many diseases, but there is no guarantee that any blood product is 100 percent free of all infectious microbes. Although it is rare, anyone who receives a blood product can be accidentally infected with an unknown pathogen.

IVIG is not generally used as a first-line therapy because of its expense and possible risks, but if you have tried other therapies for your neuropathy without seeing improvement and you can afford it, talk with your doctor about IVIG to see if you are a candidate for the treatment. For some, it makes a big difference in their neuropathy and overall health.

Immunotherapy: Take Control of Your Immune System

As you have learned throughout *The Lyme Solution*, in chronic Lyme, one of the biggest issues is an overactive immune system. When your immune system is overly reactive, it reacts to things that are otherwise benign. Allergies to foods, mold, pollen, animals, and chemical sensitivities all start to appear after exposure to Lyme disease. The Lyme organism has shifted the immune system so that your tolerance to the world around you has changed.

In conventional medicine in the United States, allergy is strictly defined. It refers to immune reactions that occur shortly after exposure to an allergen. Such immune reactions produce mild symptoms that range from sneezing, runny nose, itchy ears, and scratchy throat to more serious symptoms like hives, swollen lips, and difficulty breathing. An antibody called immunoglobulin E, or IgE, typically triggers these reactions. Although conventional medicine typically focuses on IgE responses, they are just the tip of the iceberg. The human immune system is extremely complex, and other types of immune reactions that do not involve IgE can also cause allergy-like symptoms. As a result, the non-IgE-induced symptoms may not appear for hours to days. This delay makes these other reactions harder to identify. No one test measures your response to all allergens. You and your doctor may need to use different methods to figure out which things bother you most.

As an environmental medicine physician, I am trained to examine how your surroundings affect your health. Understanding and addressing immune function in all its complexity is core to this method. That's why environmental medical practice includes additional treatments that are not in the tool kit of conventional doctors. Key interventions are the various forms of immune therapy (immunotherapy) that alter how your immune system reacts to different allergens. They give you better control over your immune system, freeing you to more efficiently defend against infection. If you have Lyme, it is essential to address allergies, because they function as immune distractions that make it harder to get rid of Lyme disease and other infections.

Now, let's delve into the treatment itself. Immunotherapy alters how your immune system reacts to any given allergic substance. Once you ascertain the substances to which you are allergic or sensitive, there are various methods to desensitize you to those specific allergens. Small amounts of the offending substances can be either injected into your skin or placed under your tongue on a daily to weekly basis. As time goes on, the amount of the substance is increased up to a maintenance dose as your immune tolerance improves. Ultimately, you can get to the point where you are no longer allergic to the material and immunotherapy can be discontinued.

There are several different types of immunotherapy. Conventional allergists usually offer injections under the skin, called *subcutaneous immunotherapy*, also known as allergy shots. This type of therapy requires doctor visits one to two times per week for up to six months to receive the shots, with the dose of allergen increased for each injection. Once you have reached your maintenance dose, you continue to get your shots every three to four weeks thereafter, which can go on for up to seven to nine years. For many people, allergy shots are inconvenient since they require going to the doctor several times per month. There is also a very small risk of developing a serious life-threatening reaction to the injections, such as swelling in your airway that stops you from breathing. The risk of developing a life-threatening reaction during an allergy shot is less than 1 percent, but it does exist.[30] Most insurance companies cover this therapy, which can reduce your sensitivity to the allergies that bother you.

Although allergy shots are a standard treatment in the United States, other approaches can also desensitize you to your allergies. The treatments I cover in this next section do not require frequent visits to the doctor. Yet they are as effective as or more effective than allergy shots.

Sublingual Immunotherapy (SLIT): How to Treat Your Allergies Drop by Drop

Although sublingual immunotherapy (SLIT) is not well known in the United States, it has been widely used throughout Europe for decades.[31] In SLIT, in place of allergy shots, doctors make highly diluted amounts of the different allergens that have been previously identified as problematic for you. Every day, a few drops of the extract are placed under the tongue. Once your extract is prescribed, you can then follow through on the treatment in the comfort of your own home. SLIT works exactly like injections—it builds immune tolerance against the allergen. Immunotherapy functions by introducing the allergen to dendritic cells, which are part of the immune system. Dendritic cells are found in the skin but also inside our mouths and under the tongue. These dendritic cells set off an immune system chain of events that alters how your body responds to an allergen.

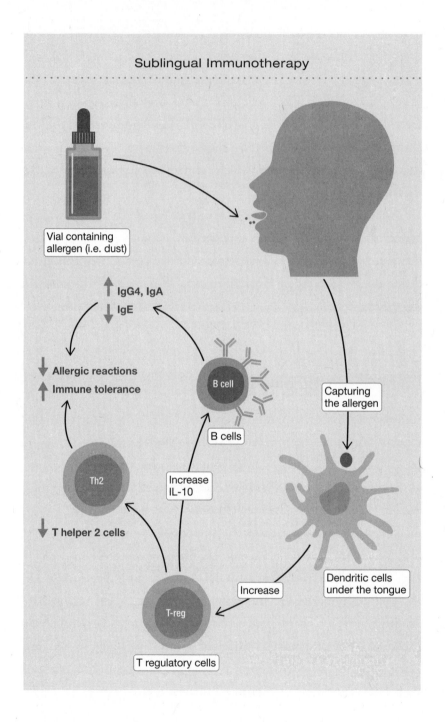

Sublingual Immunotherapy

Vial containing allergen (i.e. dust)

↑ IgG4, IgA
↓ IgE

↓ Allergic reactions
↑ Immune tolerance

B cell

B cells

Increase IL-10

Th2

↓ T helper 2 cells

Capturing the allergen

Dendritic cells under the tongue

Increase

T-reg

T regulatory cells

Over time, the reactivity to the allergen steadily decreases. This method is highly effective for control and elimination of allergies and sensitivities to foods, mold, pollen, dust, animal dander, and other allergens.

Sublingual immunotherapy has been researched extensively, with more than three hundred clinical trials and more than eight hundred studies published in the medical literature.[32] It has been in use since the early 1900s to treat mold and pollen allergies in farmers. Studies of both children and adults found SLIT to be very safe in both groups. Reports of severe allergic reaction to the treatment are extremely rare. Side effects are minimal. In many countries throughout Europe, it is the preferred method of allergy treatment because of its efficacy and lower cost.[33]

David Morris, MD, of La Crosse, Wisconsin, brought SLIT to the United States back in the 1960s. He and his group have since published several papers on the effectiveness of SLIT.[34] In fact, he was so successful with SLIT that he stopped giving allergy shots altogether in his clinic in 1972. Many people for whom allergy shots did not work well responded much better to SLIT. Unfortunately, SLIT is not approved by the Food and Drug Administration in the United States, and so many insurance companies do not reimburse for the treatment. SLIT can cost anywhere from $50 to $250 per month depending on where you live and how many allergens you are being treated for.

SLIT can be carefully customized to each individual's needs. Given the sensitivity and reactivity of those with chronic Lyme disease, this is very helpful. Doctors can adjust the dose and attune the concentration and frequency of administering the drops to your specific response. Some people are very sensitive and need smaller doses, whereas other people can tolerate much higher amounts. For example, you may need to take one to two drops up to three or four times per day. Typically, you start with a small amount and increase the dose over time until you reach a maintenance dose. SLIT allows the physician to make sure everyone gets his or her optimal dose. Many people start to feel improvement within six weeks of starting SLIT, so it doesn't take a long time to figure out whether it works for you. Treatment can last anywhere from six months to several years, so be prepared to be in it for the long haul.

People with Lyme disease often observe dramatic improvement in their symptoms with SLIT. It is one of the few therapies that induces a permanent change in the immune system and makes it stronger. While you will have to remember to take your drops every day, the investment in your health is worth it. Shifting your immune system away from the autoimmune dominant state will alleviate many of your Lyme symptoms and improve your overall immune health. The American Academy of Environmental Medicine trains doctors in SLIT treatment. Visit aaemonline.org to find a physician near you.

Low-Dose Immunotherapy (LDI): A Promising Novel Therapy

My good friend Ty Vincent, MD, of Kona, Hawaii, noticed the parallel between how the immune system reacts to Lyme and how it reacts to allergens. As I've discussed in previous chapters, through a process called *molecular mimicry*, the immune system becomes confused by microbes that resemble the molecules in our own organs and cells. Even after the organism is eradicated, the immune system is already sensitized to your own bodily tissues. Therefore, the immune reaction continues, even though the infection has cleared.

Dr. Vincent applied the principles of immunotherapy to a microbe instead of to an allergen and developed low-dose immunotherapy (LDI). In immunotherapy, the basic mechanism is to gradually reduce your reactivity to a substance by exposure to it. This, in effect, reeducates the immune system, exactly what is needed when the immune system is overreacting. In place of using an allergen as the triggering agent, Dr. Vincent used highly diluted amounts of dead microbe. He then administered the resulting treatment under the tongue, as doctors do in SLIT. He discovered that following LDI treatment, many people with Lyme significantly reduced their symptoms. When I followed his example and started using LDI, I got similar results. You will need to work with a physician who has experience with LDI, as there are many nuances to this treatment that need to be closely managed.

When the dilution is right, improvement can be seen within twenty-four to forty-eight hours. Some people experience drastic changes in their energy, neuropathy, joint or muscle pain, headaches, and sleep pattern after LDI. I've given myself LDI and noticed an almost immediate improvement in brain fog. Treatment doses are typically given every seven to eight weeks once the target dose is found, not daily as with other Lyme treatments. From the person's perspective, this is a relatively easy therapy to do. Booster doses (which are slightly weaker dilutions) can be given in between regular doses if symptoms start to return. While the upsides of LDI are obvious, it can sometimes take a little work to find your target dose because it varies from person to person—so you may not see any change with your first few doses. Your doctor will usually start with a weak dilution and move on to stronger dilutions if there is no change with the previous treatment.

There is one more significant disadvantage of LDI. If the dose given is too strong, it can cause Lyme symptoms to flare. Although those of us who do LDI do all we can to prevent this, it does happen occasionally. It is similar to having a Herx reaction when you are actively treating Lyme disease. Although the reaction can be uncomfortable, it confirms that the organism being treated is part of what causes your symptoms. Fortunately, most of these types of reactions are short-lived. Plus, they quickly help doctors to fine-tune the ideal dose.

My colleagues who use LDI report good results. Based on this clinical experience, doctors like me know that LDI has helped many people with Lyme disease. It seems to be effective for people who have either acute or chronic Lyme disease, so it doesn't matter where you are in your illness. It can be used with people who have done numerous rounds of antibiotics, herbs, and other Lyme treatments. It still works in most cases. If you have tried other approaches and are still struggling, this treatment may very well be the missing piece in your journey.

GWEN'S STORY

Gwen was referred to me by one of my functional medicine colleagues. She had been battling Lyme disease for more than a year and had consulted a few well-known Lyme doctors around the country. As typically happens, they had put her on several courses of antibiotics. Her primary complaints were brain fog, fatigue, and severe bloating. She did not have typical Lyme disease and, fortunately, did not have any joint or muscle issues. Gwen told me that every time she took antibiotics, her stomach felt terrible and her bloating got worse. She said she always looked seven months pregnant. On more than one occasion, she'd been asked when she was due.

Gwen began the Immune-Boosting Diet immediately. She next took a stool test to ascertain whether she had any underlying infection. Her stool test was negative. As the diet alkalinized her system, I put her on a course of Chinese herbs and other nutritional supplements to improve her intestinal function. After a month, her bloating and fatigue were better. However, her persistent brain fog interfered with her work as a graphic designer. I started Gwen on low-dose immunotherapy. After ten days, she called and told me she felt better for five days, but then her symptoms returned. A booster dose helped reduce her symptoms until the next treatment. Over the course of the series of treatment, Gwen's energy improved, and her bloating subsided. The brain fog persisted longer than her other symptoms. Since then, Gwen has seen me for an additional five doses of the bimonthly Lyme LDI treatment. With each treatment, her relief from symptoms has lasted longer and longer. At this point, it has been over four months since her last treatment. Gwen no longer experiences fatigue, brain fog, or bloating. She has been able to stop the herbal protocol. She is now able to maintain her health with an alkaline diet and regular exercise.

Low-Dose Naltrexone

Naltrexone is a prescription medication traditionally used to treat alcohol and narcotic addiction. It works by blocking opioid receptors in the brain, which curtails the cravings for these addictive substances. However, researchers have discovered that when naltrexone is used at very low doses, it has an immune-modulating effect and reduces pain. More than ninety published studies document the efficacy of low-dose naltrexone (LDN) for various illnesses including Crohn's disease, fibromyalgia, multiple sclerosis, depression, cancer, and other autoimmune diseases.[35]

LDN has several known mechanisms of action. Its better-known mechanism causes the brain to release more of your own natural painkillers. This makes it particularly useful in treating pain without using harmful steroids or anti-inflammatory medications. LDN also seems to reduce inflammation in the brain, which thereby reduces pain, but may also improve cognitive function and neuropathy. Many people with Lyme disease who use LDN experience better sleep, improved brain function, reduced joint or muscle aches, better bowel function, and more energy.

Considered an experimental treatment for this purpose, LDN is used off-label. Naltrexone was originally developed to treat drug and alcohol abuse but is used at much higher doses for those purposes. LDN has an excellent safety record and is generally very well tolerated. When they start LDN therapy, some people report that they experience insomnia, vivid dreams, or anxiety. If your doctor starts you on lower doses, this rarely happens. LDN is a prescription medicine, so you will need to work with your doctor. Since it is used off-label, insurance does not usually pay for it, but it is very inexpensive, so most people can afford it. Take 1 milligram at bedtime and increase by 1 milligram every two weeks if there is no improvement in symptoms. Most women do best at 3 milligrams at night and men often do best at 4.5 milligrams nightly. However, LDN has virtually no toxicity, so higher doses can be tried if needed.

Homeopathy: When Less Is More

Homeopathy is a centuries-old system of medicine founded by Samuel Hahnemann, MD, in 1796. Homeopathic remedies are highly diluted substances derived from plant, animal, or mineral sources that stimulate the body's natural healing ability. Homeopathy's foundational concept is that "like cures like." It seeks to correct health issues experienced in a symptomatic person by introducing substances that would normally cause the very same symptoms in a healthy person. For example, drinking strong coffee can cause heart palpitations, restlessness, insomnia, and shakiness in an average, healthy person. So a homeopath may prescribe homeopathic coffee (*Coffea cruda*) for someone who complains of having these same symptoms that are not occasioned by consuming coffee.

When a homeopath selects a remedy, he or she considers the totality of that individual's symptoms—physical, mental, and emotional. Each one of ten people who experience a similar symptom will very likely receive an entirely different remedy, based on a range of factors that differ from person to person. For example, each person with a headache may have experienced its onset at a different time of day, or may have diverse accompanying symptoms, such as nausea, pressure at the neck, or other distinguishing differences. I like homeopathy because it is a safe, effective treatment for many people with Lyme disease. Although I improved dramatically with herbs in healing my own Lyme, it was my homeopath who got me 100 percent symptom-free.

Homeopathy is widely used throughout the world, especially in India, South America, and parts of Europe, but has not been as popular in the United States. In the conventional medical community, there has been controversy about it since its exact mechanism of action is unknown at present. Nonetheless, research and a long history of clinical use have found homeopathy to be safe and effective for people of any age. It is also one of the few medical treatments that truly addresses the whole person. You may find that your local health food store sells homeopathic remedies, but I do not recommend self-treating. Homeopathic practitioners spend years studying the more than two thousand remedies in use, so trying to treat yourself would be looking for a needle in a stack of needles. This is best left in the hands of a professional who can properly analyze your case and give you the best remedy. See the Resources section (page 325) for a list of homeopathic practitioners.

Your Doctor as Your Partner

Using the more advanced options in this chapter requires building a good relationship with your physician or health-care provider. Anyone can safely follow the Five-Stage Immune-Boosting Plan detailed in Part Two of this book. However, for those who still need to access the advanced therapies, you must consult a professional. Find someone you work well with, who will be an advocate for your health and well-being. Too many doctors out there can be dismissive of your symptoms—and some of them may be downright antagonistic toward you. When you are sick and not feeling well, it's hard to have the energy to fight. You spend countless hours on the Internet trying to figure out what the next step might be. You are exhausted trying to piece together your plan of action. I know because I've been there.

But here's the thing. You don't have to do this alone. Fortunately, there are naturopaths, medical doctors, nurses, physician assistants, nurse practitioners, chiropractors, and others who are on your side. One of the biggest issues with Lyme is that people are often anxious to move on to the next treatment when they haven't given the current one a chance to work. At some level, you need to trust whomever you are working with. If you don't, then it's best to find someone you do trust who is a better fit for you. It is a tremendous relief when you have a captain of your ship, guiding the way, versus having to figure it all out on your own.

When I meet with someone, I hope to establish a partnership where we are both equally invested in getting you well again. A third tenet of naturopathic medicine is *Docere*, or "doctor as teacher." A large part of my job is to educate you on what you can do to repair and restore your body to better health. The body has the capacity to heal—you just need to give it the right tools to do so. You and your provider need to have a therapeutic relationship, one where he or she provides guidance and support for your physical, mental, and emotional well-being. If you haven't found the right person yet, reach out to others in your local community and find out whom they recommend. Or check the Resources section (page 325), which lists people I know and trust to provide the support you need.

CHAPTER 9

Am I Better? How to Cycle Back Through the Five-Stage Plan If You're Not

A question people with Lyme disease frequently ask is "How will I know if I'm better?" The simple answer is that you'll know when your symptoms improve, when all of the problems that have plagued you since you were bitten by a tick start to go away. The more complicated—and realistic—answer is that you will finally start to have more good days than bad. There is no unilateral trajectory toward healing. The process is almost never that consistent. You will have ups and downs—some good days and some bad days. Many people get discouraged, making it essential that you change your mind-set. Rather than expect a quick total cure, pay attention to how you feel week by week and month by month. It's important to remember that the lab tests for Lyme disease will not accurately tell you or your doctor how you're doing (see Chapter 2). At the end of the day, the way you feel is the best measurement of the effectiveness of your treatment.

Progress can be slow and easy to take for granted. To keep track of how far you've come, keep a symptom journal. Or retake the Lyme Disease Symptom Questionnaire (page 42) periodically to follow your evolving improvement. When you are not feeling well, your goal will always be to feel 100 percent better. When there is only 50 percent improvement and you still have more work to do, it is easy to dismiss the real progress you have made.

As people get better, it's natural to forget many of the symptoms that have slowly gone away since they were first diagnosed. Suppose someone complained of headaches, joint pain, and fatigue. When, three months later, the headaches and joint pain have disappeared, it's easy to overfocus on the persistent fatigue. Nevertheless, the lessening of any symptoms is real progress, although it may not seem that way today when the fatigue is most bothersome.

When I was a child growing up in Southern California, one of my favorite Disneyland activities was Mr. Toad's Wild Ride. You climb aboard and head in a certain direction. When an obstacle looms up before you, at the last minute, you make a sharp turn in a different direction. For many people with Lyme disease, healing from Lyme resembles a wild ride. Things are going reasonably well when, at the blink of an eye, you find yourself having symptoms again for no apparent reason. This can be frustrating, discouraging, irritating, and even depressing. I used to get flare-ups of neuropathy early in my Lyme process and would worry every time that my Lyme disease was getting worse. I finally noticed that specific triggers were causing them, such as coffee, stress, and lack of sleep, and if I avoided or controlled these triggers, I felt fine. While not everyone can easily figure out what sets their symptoms off, it is worth looking at what you are doing in your life that may make your symptoms worse.

If you have already been through *The Lyme Solution* program and are still having symptoms, you may be asking yourself, "Now what?" You must be honest with yourself about whether you have truly done all the hard work necessary to get well—work that entails following the diet, taking the herbs, and making the lifestyle changes in this book. Doing all of that is not easy. It takes time and effort to overhaul your life and to break patterns you established as a child.

But remember, the choices you make affect your health. I know firsthand. I love coffee, but when I drink it, my neuropathy gets worse. You have to decide for yourself what you are willing to sacrifice in order to completely recover.

Face up to the truth. If, for example, you have not been disciplined in following the program, go back and try again. Be diligent with each of the recommendations. You'll find more success when you do. If you have followed the program thoroughly and you are still feeling stuck, then it may be time to start looking at other possibilities.

Lab Tests That Matter

As you read in Chapter 2, lab tests for Lyme are not that useful in monitoring your progress in treating Lyme disease. Nevertheless, certain additional types of lab tests can ensure that you (or your doctor) have not missed other non-Lyme reasons why you feel unwell. Additional lab tests can also give you insight into how your body functions. You will need to work with your health-care provider to have these lab tests run. Here are some I recommend:

Inflammation

If you continue to have joint or muscle pain, headaches, abdominal pain, or swelling in your hands or feet, you can be tested for other possible causes. Several blood tests measure bodily levels of inflammation. On most of the following tests, people with Lyme tend to show a normal result, so when the lab results are elevated, there may be something else going on.

C-REACTIVE PROTEIN (CRP) TEST

In response to inflammation anywhere in the body, the liver produces this protein. As such, when a test shows elevated CRP levels, it can be due to causes such as bacterial infections to autoimmune disease, heart disease, or cancer. Because CRP is a nonspecific marker, high levels don't tell you specifically what is wrong. But a high level does reveal that something is aggravating your immune system and can prompt your doctor to look for other causes. A CRP level greater than 10 mg/L almost always indicates a bacterial infection.

ERYTHROCYTE SEDIMENTATION RATE (ESR) TEST

Often used to screen for inflammation, this inexpensive test is another nonspecific measurement of inflammation. However, the ESR can also be affected by noninflammatory factors such as pregnancy and use of certain medications. Nonetheless, the low cost and ease of use make it useful in monitoring inflammation.

INFLAMMATORY CYTOKINES TEST

Cytokines are the chemicals that allow immune cells to talk to each other. Some of these substances promote inflammation, while others turn inflammation off. Cytokines perform many other functions to fight infection. Research shows that patients with early Lyme disease have high levels of proinflammatory cytokines, such as interleukin-1 (IL-1) and tumor necrosis factor-alpha (TNF-α).[1] The downside to testing cytokines is that their presence in the bloodstream can be very short lived, so they can be difficult to detect. But if you have active inflammation, these tests can help get to the source of the problem.

In summary, all of these tests are available from most labs your doctor would use. They can be part of an initial Lyme disease workup, or to look into inflammation and monitor efficacy at any point in your treatment. These tests may also give your doctor an idea if there is something else going on with you other than Lyme disease. If the treatment plan for Lyme (or other causes) works, these inflammatory markers will go down and become normal.

Immune Status

Since the immune system is so complex, no one blood test can measure how well it's working. However, many patients with Lyme disease show abnormalities on certain immune tests. All of the following signify that your immune system may not be up to par:

- If you get sick all the time
- If you pick up every cold that comes your way
- If your health as a child was poor
- If you regularly miss school or work

Testing your immune system, through any of the following tests, can tell you if you were born with an immune problem or perhaps acquired one later in life.

COMPLETE BLOOD COUNT (CBC)

Part of every routine health checkup, a complete blood count (CBC) examines both white and red blood cells. Elevated white-blood-cell counts suggest infection. *Neutrophils* (one type of white blood cell) increase with bacterial infections. *Lymphocytes* (another type of white blood cell) rise with viral infections. Ironically, some viruses will actually cause your white blood cell count to go down. HIV is the most well known, but other viruses like Epstein-Barr, influenza, or cold viruses can also cause the white blood cell count to drop. Since white blood cells fight infection, lower numbers of them compromise the immune system and make it more difficult to fight off infection, including Lyme disease.

IMMUNOGLOBULINS

As I've mentioned earlier, immunoglobulins are antibodies that identify and eliminate unwanted microbes. Our bodies make five different types of antibodies: IgG, IgM, IgA, IgE, and IgD. The three most important for fighting infection are IgG, IgM, and IgA (IgE is linked to allergic reactions, and IgD is produced in such small quantities that its significance is unknown). Deficiencies in any of these antibodies can make it harder to fight off infection effectively. IgM is found in the blood exclusively, whereas IgG and IgA can be found in both the blood and tissue.

You can either inherit or acquire immune deficiencies, but in both cases they may lead to chronic immune problems. Many of the blood tests used to diagnose infection look for elevated antibodies, which indicates the body is fighting off the intruders. But since people with immune deficiencies don't produce enough antibodies, they may receive a false negative test result.

C4A COMPLEMENT

C4a complement is a part of your immune system that boosts the effects of antibodies in eliminating microbes. Complement binds to the surface of a microbe and punches holes in its cell membrane, ultimately destroying it. Complement is actually a sequence of proteins that is activated by certain antibodies. The antibodies set off the proteins like a series of stacked dominoes, with one protein setting off the next. One of the by-products is called C4a, which occurs early in the cascade. Research shows that patients with acute Lyme disease have elevated levels of C3a and C4a, but those with chronic Lyme disease, with primarily joint and muscle symptoms, have only increased C4a blood amounts.[2] This test can be useful during the active treatment phase to make sure the therapy is working effectively.

TRANSFORMING GROWTH FACTOR-β_1 (TGF-β_1)

Secreted by most white blood cells, this molecule is partially responsible for controlling the immune system. Studies show that TGF-β_1 increases in patients with early Lyme disease but goes down in those with chronic Lyme disease.[3] I sometimes use this test to follow the course of treatment, especially for people with initially elevated TGF-β_1 levels. This test is also elevated in those with mold toxicity, so it can be useful in monitoring mold treatment as well.

Since each of these cells contributes to immune function, low amounts can suggest an inability to fight infection. These tests measure blood levels of T cells, B cells, and natural killer (NK) cells to ascertain if there is any deficiency. Many people with Lyme disease have a low count of NK cells (CD57 cells), which are direct scavengers of infection. While a low NK cell count is not specific to Lyme disease, this test can be helpful during treatment to see if your immune system is improving.

Our knowledge about the immune system is still in its infancy. We are still trying to learn how it functions and find new ways to measure how it works. Technology has not yet advanced to the point of providing better functional tests of the immune system. However, for some people with Lyme disease, these tests can indicate how to change the direction of treatment or pinpoint where there may be a deficit.

Nutritional Status

We who live in the United States or other modern, industrialized countries rarely think about malnutrition or nutritional deficiencies. Our image of malnutrition may come from late-night television commercials showing starving children in Africa with large, distended bellies. That's why many Americans are surprised to learn that malnutrition and poor absorption are so common in the modern world.[4] The varied reasons that Americans may experience malnutrition include the following:

- Consumption of highly processed foods stripped of their nutrients

- Consumption of foods tainted with nutrient-depleting presti-cides
- Gastrointestinal problems that interfere with the ability to absorb nutrients

I always inquire into every patient's diet, eating habits, quality of food (organic versus nonorganic), and meal patterns. I also ask about their digestive function and history of intestinal disease. Each of these factors reveals how the patient is digesting and absorbing their food, as well as uncovering the diversity and quality of their diet. As mentioned earlier, many people with Lyme disease eat a standard American diet, consisting of low-quality processed foods that lack vital nutrients.

If you have not gotten the treatment results you want, please recommit to following the Immune-Boosting Diet. Given the brain fog that sometimes accompanies Lyme disease, many people find it helpful to keep a diet diary so that they can see what they actually eat—and where they can improve their nutrition. Write down everything you eat and drink for five days, and review it to figure out where to make changes.

Even if you eat a whole-foods, organic diet, it's advisable to check out how well your body assimilates your food. Unfortunately, the best way to measure this is to take a tissue sample from fat or muscle, but because this is so invasive, it's not routinely done. However, doctors can still get a relatively good idea of your nutritional status from specific blood tests. These tests include the following:

RED BLOOD CELL ELEMENTS

Measuring the amount of vitamins or minerals inside your red blood cells gives a close approximation of what may be in your tissues. Since red blood cells stay in your body for about three months, they are themselves a type of tissue cell. You can also measure vitamins and minerals from a regular blood sample, but some nutrients fluctuate so much in the blood that a single measurement may not accurately reflect what is inside your cells. For example, B vitamins, because they are water-soluble, are not stored in the body, so your blood levels of B vitamins would be greatly affected by recent dietary intake or by taking a nutritional supplement that contains them. But overall, measuring red blood cell elements is fairly accurate in revealing your long-term nutritional status.

AMINO ACIDS

Amino acids are the building blocks of protein, involved in making neurotransmitters, building muscle, and producing energy. They act as precursors to hormones, including thyroid hormone. Either lack of protein or decreased ability to break down protein can lead to amino acid deficiencies. Some amino acids are called *essential*, which means your body cannot make them on its own. These are histidine, isoleucine, leucine, lysine, methionine, phenylalanine, threonine, tryptophan, and valine. The body can manufacture the other amino acids. Both blood and urine tests can measure amino acids. I use two tests: blood amino acid testing to measure essential amino acids, and a twenty-four-hour urine amino acid test to assess whether the body is effectively metabolizing amino acids. Many patients with Lyme disease have deficiencies in amino acids, so these tests identify whether your protein intake is sufficient, or if your body is wasting protein too quickly. The twenty-four-hour urine amino acid test is better at detecting early deficiency than blood testing.

IRON

Your body uses iron to make hemoglobin, which carries oxygen to your tissues. Iron forms a part of each red blood cell, so iron deficiency can lead to anemia. Iron is also necessary for thyroid metabolism, so low iron levels can impair your body's ability to make active thyroid hormone. Iron deficiency has been associated with fatigue, restless legs syndrome, muscle weakness, brittle nails, pale skin, dizziness, headaches, and cold hands or feet. Women are more prone to iron deficiency due to blood loss during their menstrual cycle. Chronic infection, like Lyme disease, can cause iron levels to drop. However, don't eat more iron-rich foods or take an iron supplement if you don't need to. One of the most common genetically inherited diseases is hemochromatosis, in which the body stores iron to toxic levels. People with this condition need to be very careful with their iron intake.

To measure iron levels, your doctor can run an iron profile, which includes measurement of serum iron and ferritin. Ferritin is the protein that stores iron in almost all living organisms. Ferritin usually drops when you become iron deficient, even before blood levels of iron have changed. This is more common in women but can occur in men, too. If you need iron, taking vitamin C with your iron supplement can increase absorption. Foods rich in iron include red meat, organ meats, dark-green leafy vegetables, nuts and seeds, beans, and blackstrap molasses. Coffee, tea, soy, and calcium products all block the absorption of iron, so do not take your iron supplement within thirty minutes of eating these foods. Consume them cautiously as well, if you want to increase your iron stores.

VITAMIN D

Vitamin D is a hormone rather than a true vitamin. It's an immune modulator. That means that it helps regulate immune function by either strengthening or weakening an immune response as needed. Almost all of bodily vitamin D comes from unblocked sun exposure—little is obtained from diet. I recommend measuring 25-hydroxy vitamin D to ensure you are getting adequate amounts of vitamin D. Try to get your blood level between 40 and 100 ng/mL. According to the Vitamin D Council, 40 ng/mL is the minimum before you start running into health problems.[5] If you are deficient, then increase your sun exposure or take a vitamin D supplement to increase your vitamin D levels.

SELECT NUTRIENTS

In order to optimize nutrient levels, you must consume—and be able to digest and absorb—a variety of foods. Certain specific nutrients are more critical than others. As part of troubleshooting to improve your treatment results, it's often helpful to ask your doctor to check for deficiencies of specific nutrients. I recommend checking blood levels of coenzyme Q10, carnitine, or fatty acids, for example, if appropriate for people who may have undiagnosed nutrient deficiencies. Your nutritionally oriented doctor can help you determine if these tests are necessary.

What do test results reveal? Labs typically compare your results with those in the so-called reference range, which is a particular nutrient's range of levels in the blood of a healthy person. But note that the reference range with a blood test reflects where the general population falls, not necessarily what is optimal for you. There has never been good research to define what levels are best for each age group and gender. As a general rule, blood nutrient concentrations should be at least at the upper end of the normal range. If you are supplementing with any nutrient, ask your doctor to repeat the lab tests every three to six months to make sure your levels have increased as expected. You can then modify your dose accordingly.

Intestinal Function

As I mentioned earlier in this book, your intestinal tract accounts for up to 80 percent of your immune function. Your gut is where most of your healthy microbes live. That's why gut health is a key factor in getting well. If you continue experiencing constipation, diarrhea, abdominal pain, indigestion, reflux, gas, or bloating, even after following my Immune-Boosting Gut Protocol, it's possible that an underlying problem is in your gut. If you have previously been or are currently on antibiotics, you have no doubt altered your normal gut flora. Further investigation of your stomach and intestinal function will identify the causes of your symptoms.

Gastroenterologists commonly use endoscopy or colonoscopy to look down the throat into the stomach or up the colon. While these procedures are good at identifying tumors, polyps, ulcers, or other types of inflammation, they don't assess gut function. Even routine stool testing looks only at common bacterial infections or food poisoning.

COMPREHENSIVE STOOL ANALYSIS

To better evaluate gut function, some specialty labs offer a more comprehensive stool analysis that measures various aspects of digestion and inflammation. The analysis includes these tests:

- Bacterial growth. This test measures both normal and abnormal bacterial growth.
- Yeast culture. Some yeast in the stool is normal. But yeast can often overgrow in the intestines after antibiotic treatment. This test checks for an abnormal overgrowth of different types of yeast.
- Parasite identification. This looks at hidden parasite infection.
- Secretory IgA. This test measures a deficiency or an increase in IgA (immunoglobulin A), which can suggest underlying illness in the gut. Immunoglobulin A lines all of your mucous membranes.
- Digestive markers. These measure how well your body is breaking down protein, carbohydrates, and fats. Deficiencies in these enzymes can lead to food allergies or other gastrointestinal problems.
- Inflammatory markers. Increased amounts of calprotectin, lysozyme, and lactoferrin can all be associated with inflammation in the gut. Elevation in these markers can be seen with irritable bowel syndrome, Crohn's disease, ulcerative colitis, celiac disease, and infection. These can be used to monitor treatment when you are trying to reduce inflammation in your gut.
- Short-chain fatty acids. These are produced by normal, healthy bacteria, so deficiencies in these fatty acids can suggest that you do not have enough beneficial bacteria in your gut.
- Red blood cells and white blood cells. This test can show if there is internal bleeding or underlying infection.
- pH. Your beneficial bacteria thrive at a slightly alkaline pH, so a pH test is a good way to make sure you are keeping your diet alkaline. When some bacteria start to overgrow or pathogenic

bacteria invade the intestines, they can produce certain acids as by-products, which will decrease your pH. A very acidic pH can also indicate that your diet is too acidic.

A CSA reveals current gut status across this range of indicators. This provides useful information to direct treatment, so that you can pinpoint exactly which supplements you need. With the test results, your doctor will know what nutrients, probiotics, or other substances will restore your gut health. Some supplements must be avoided prior to doing this test, such as digestive enzymes and probiotics. Check with your physician to make sure you don't take anything that might interfere with the test.

HYDROGEN AND METHANE BREATH TEST

To diagnose a condition known as small-intestine bacterial overgrowth (SIBO; see the discussion later in this chapter), the doctor has the patient drink a sugar solution and then blow into a series of tubes. If the patient has abnormal bacterial growth in the small intestines, their breath will contain high amounts of either hydrogen or methane, which this test will measure. Many people with Lyme disease have this condition, perhaps due to prolonged use of antibiotics. Easy to perform, this test is indicated for anyone who has had long-standing stomach or bowel problems that don't ever seem to go away. This test can also be used to diagnose sucralase deficiency, the inability to break down table sugar (sucrose). Both SIBO and sucrase deficiency cause similar symptoms, so both tests may be necessary if you have these symptoms.

Note this important guideline for this sequence of tests: if your test results reveal abnormalities, repeat these tests following treatment, to make sure that you have repaired any damage to the gut and restored your normal intestinal flora. Treatment can take up to six months, so plan on redoing these tests at that time. If there is any sign of bleeding, talk with your doctor or gastroenterologist to make sure there is nothing more serious affecting your gut.

Metabolic Function

Unless you work with a Lyme-literate doctor, the hormonal and metabolic problems that often accompany Lyme disease may be overlooked. Quite often, Lyme disease affects the hormone system, especially the thyroid. As I discussed in Chapter 7, an underactive thyroid leads to symptoms like persistent fatigue, inadequate sleep, weight gain, constipation, worse allergic symptoms, or poor immune function. If you experience any of these symptoms, ask your doctor to run the tests listed in this section. In my practice, as many as 40 percent of my patients with Lyme disease also have an underactive thyroid. Many of them tell me their thyroid problems began after they were bitten by a tick. Of those with a slow-functioning thyroid, the majority have Hashimoto's thyroiditis, which is an autoimmune form of hypothyroidism. While this does not prove cause and effect, it certainly makes me suspicious that Lyme disease is the cause of their thyroid problems. Other doctors I know who treat Lyme disease have observed the same problem. My good friend Amy Myers, MD, *New York Times* best-selling author of *The Autoimmune Solution* and *The Thyroid Connection*, describes in her latest book how infection can trigger autoimmune thyroid problems. Several microbes are capable of causing thyroid problems, and Lyme happens to be one of them.

Many people with Lyme disease develop blood sugar abnormalities and become insulin resistant. Here's what frequently happens: it's normal for the body to make insulin, a hormone needed to transport glucose into your cells. Insulin resistance occurs when the body's cells fail to respond to insulin, so sugar can't get into the cells and continues to increase in the blood. Also known as *metabolic syndrome*, insulin resistance acts as a precursor to diabetes. Early in the condition, people with insulin resistance have few or no symptoms but can go on to develop fatigue, weight gain, or skin tags or dark patches of skin on the back of the neck, groin, and armpit, called *acanthosis nigricans*. Women with insulin resistance are at greater risk of developing obesity, diabetes, heart disease, breast or uterine cancer, and polycystic ovarian syndrome (PCOS).

Work with your doctor to make sure you are metabolically and hormonally balanced. Your primary-care provider can order most of these tests, but you may want to see an endocrinologist if you need more specific testing. Some labs I regularly run include the following:

COMPREHENSIVE METABOLIC PROFILE

This routine blood test, which every lab in the world performs, looks at blood sugar, electrolytes, liver function, kidney function, fluid balance, and protein. This is a quick, easy way to make sure that no obvious underlying disease is making you sick.

THYROID FUNCTION TESTS

This battery of tests includes thyroid-stimulating hormone (TSH), free T3, free T4, and thyroid antibodies. T3 and T4 are produced in the thyroid gland and are the hormones that stimulate your metabolism. Most doctors run only TSH, but on its own, this test can miss early thyroid disease. I have seen patients with positive thyroid antibodies *before* there are changes in TSH. Thyroid antibodies can be produced if an autoimmune process is attacking the thyroid, so it is important to check that none are present. Otherwise, it's like watching a train that is about to wreck. I prefer to intervene before the train crashes.

ADRENAL FUNCTION TESTS

In people with Lyme disease, three important hormones made by the adrenal gland may also be affected. Although each hormone serves a different purpose, low levels of these hormones can make you feel tired, dizzy, and unbalanced.

Cortisol is the most important adrenal hormone affected by Lyme disease. This hormone has a specific rhythm: it's at its peak early in the morning and goes down as the day progresses. To get the most accurate measurement, therefore, the blood test for cortisol should be done between six a.m. and eight a.m. You'll see that the reference range is very wide for this test (between 7 and 28 mcg/dL.) Most people feel better when their cortisol levels are at the higher end of that range.

Do you find that you always crave salt? Or do you become dizzy or light-headed every time you stand up? These may be signs that you have low aldosterone. *Aldosterone* is another adrenal hormone that controls salt metabolism and blood pressure. If your blood pressure is always low, it can be a sign of low aldosterone. Aldosterone is rarely low in people with Lyme disease, but I have seen it.

DHEA is the third adrenal hormone. DHEA levels peak during your early twenties and then slowly decline with age. I measure DHEA if indicated. Men nearly always have higher levels of DHEA than women, so women are more susceptible to having symptoms such as fatigue, hair loss, low strength and stamina, and low libido as DHEA starts to drop. I always check DHEA-sulfate, as this is the more stable form of DHEA in the blood.

ORGANIC ACID TEST (OAT)

Run by several specialty labs, this nutritional test measures metabolites related to gastrointestinal, cellular, and mitochondrial function, as well as neurotransmitter balance. This test casts a wide net to pick up subtle alterations in metabolism. Organic acids are naturally produced as a by-product of metabolism, so increases or deficits in specific acids can show where imbalances exist. Many imbalances can be corrected through diet and nutrition, so the OAT test results will help you and your doctor focus your treatment.

GENETIC TESTS

Two levels of genetic tests are currently available. The most popular type is the test for single nucleotide polymorphisms (SNPs). These small mutations occurring in the genetic code can alter how that specific gene functions. Although there are more than ten million SNPs in the average human, most have no adverse effect on health. However, some do. Some SNPs can predict how your body reacts when exposed to a certain toxin or drug, what disease you may be at most risk of developing, or how your body metabolizes certain nutrients.

Many physicians look more closely at an individual's genes to determine the best treatments, or what treatments should be avoided. The downside is that SNP testing is not conclusive: having a certain SNP does not necessarily mean that the gene associated with it fails to function properly. This can lead to unnecessary treatment. Unfortunately, in this case the technology is ahead of our understanding. Since everyone has SNPs, we are still to trying to comprehend which ones are most important and how to best treat people with these variations.

The second type of genetic testing is for inherited diseases. Most inherited genetic diseases show up early in life and can produce serious symptoms. Some genetic conditions do not show up until later—for example, Huntington's disease, which involves a progressive deterioration of the brain and nerves that is ultimately fatal. The good news is that these types of genetic diseases are rare. They are almost never found in people with Lyme disease. This type of testing is not needed for people with Lyme disease, unless there is a family history of one of these inherited illnesses.

People with Lyme disease do, however, commonly have metabolic and hormone issues like those I mention in this chapter. Getting these problems diagnosed may play a large part in your getting well, especially if your doctor has never looked at these aspects of your health. Once you determine exactly what is not functioning properly, you can correct metabolic issues fairly easily. After treatment is started, people start to feel better quickly. For example, thyroid metabolism is fast, so it doesn't take long to find the right dose of thyroid hormone if someone has an underactive thyroid. Correcting metabolic or hormonal imbalances can usually be done within a matter of weeks or month.

The table on the following pages contains a summary of the tests discussed in this chapter.

TYPE	TEST	WHAT DOES IT MEASURE?	WHAT DOES IT MEAN?
Inflammation	C-reactive protein (CRP)	Nonspecific	Elevated levels are sign of inflammation
	Erythrocyte sedimentation rate (ESR)	Nonspecific	Elevated levels are sign of inflammation
	Inflammatory cytokines	Cytokines	Patients with early Lyme disease have high levels of proinflammatory cytokines, such as interleukin-1 (IL-1) and tumor necrosis factor-alpha (TNF-α)[6]
Immune Status	Complete blood count (CBC)	Red and white blood cells	Elevated white blood cell count in infection; high neutrophils suggest bacterial infection, while increased lymphocytes suggests viral infection; low red cell count means anemia
	Immunoglobulins	IgG, IgM, and IgA	High amounts suggest immune activation; low levels suggest immune deficiency

TYPE	TEST	WHAT DOES IT MEASURE?	WHAT DOES IT MEAN?
Immune Status	C4a complement	C4a	Increased C4a seen in Lyme and mold-toxic people
	Transforming growth factor-β1 (TGF-β1)	TGF-β1	Also elevated in Lyme and mold toxicity
	T and B cell subsets	T cells, B cells, and NK cells	CD57 cells may be low in patients with Lyme disease
Nutritional Status	Red blood cell elements	Minerals and toxic metals, such as lead, mercury, and arsenic	Low nutrient levels suggest inadequate intake or poor absorption
	Amino acids	Amino acids from blood or urine	Low levels may mean poor intake or increased metabolism
	Iron	Serum iron and ferritin, an iron storage form	Decreased serum iron or ferritin suggests lack of intake, poor absorption, or chronic infection; high amounts can mean excess intake or hemochromatosis
	Vitamin D	Vitamin D	Low vitamin D levels are often seen in patients with Lyme disease
	Select nutrients	Specific vitamin, mineral, or other nutrient	High or low amounts reflect dietary intake and utilization

TYPE	TEST	WHAT DOES IT MEASURE?	WHAT DOES IT MEAN?
Intestinal Function	Comprehensive stool analysis	Bacteria and yeast culture, parasite analysis, digestive function, inflammatory markers, IgA, pH, blood in stool, and short-chain fatty acids	High or low levels show current state of intestinal health and digestive function
	Hydrogen and methane breath test	SIBO or sucralase deficiency	Elevated hydrogen or methane suggests an overgrowth of bacteria in small intestine or deficiency of sucralase
Metabolic Function	Comprehensive metabolic profile	Blood sugar (glucose), electrolytes, kidney function, liver function	High or low values show metabolic dysfunction, kidney disease, or liver disease
	Thyroid function tests	TSH, free T3, free T4, thyroid antibodies	High TSH, low free T3 or T4 indicate an underactive thyroid, often seen in patients with Lyme disease
	Adrenal function tests	Cortisol, aldosterone, and DHEA	Low adrenal hormones can be a sign of chronic stress or hormone imbalance

TYPE	TEST	WHAT DOES IT MEASURE?	WHAT DOES IT MEAN?
Metabolic Function	Organic acid test (OAT)	Organic acids that are breakdown products of various metabolic pathways	High or low levels show where metabolism is overactive or underactive
	Genetic tests	SNPs or inherited genetic diseases	Certain genetic mutations can suggest defects in the corresponding pathways

Other Conditions That Plague People with Lyme Disease

Once Lyme has affected you, it's easy to feel that your every symptom is Lyme-related, but that's not always so. I call this the *Lyme Black Hole*. It can be challenging for you and your doctor to avoid falling into this hole and to keep looking at other possible causes that may adversely affect your health. Just because you have Lyme disease does not mean you do not also have some other health condition that may be causing your symptoms. Following are some of the more common conditions that get missed in some people with Lyme disease:

Small Intestine Bacterial Overgrowth (SIBO)

Most of the body's beneficial bacteria live in the colon. There they do all of the following:

- Break down fiber from food
- Make B vitamins and vitamin K
- Help to eliminate harmful toxins
- Support the immune system

Doctors long believed that the small intestine was mostly sterile, with little growth of bacteria.[7] However, newer research shows that this is not entirely true—the small intestine simply harbors different kinds of bacteria than those found in the large intestine.[8] These small-intestine microbes are believed to be part of the normal flora and may protect from dangerous bacteria or parasites.

Just like the large intestine, the small intestine can also develop an overgrowth of unfriendly bacteria. This frequently happens when people overuse antibiotics. Or it may be due to another underlying condition that disposes the person to SIBO, including diabetes, Crohn's disease, or other nervous system diseases that affect gut function. If you have constant gas, bloating, diarrhea, and abdominal pain, you may have SIBO. It can also cause irregular bowel movements. Because the small intestine is where most digestion and absorption of nutrients takes place, these unusual bacteria start to inappropriately digest your food, leading to gas production and inflammatory substances that irritate your gut lining.

SIBO can go undiagnosed for years. In fact, many scientists believe it's a common cause of IBS.[9] Many patients with Lyme disease who have been on antibiotics long term or have neurological involvement that affects their bowel habits can develop IBS. As mentioned earlier, a simple hydrogen and methane breath test can diagnose this problem. Elevated levels of hydrogen or methane found in the breath strongly suggest SIBO. There are many different ways of treating

SIBO. Conventional doctors often prescribe antibiotics, specifically rifaximin or neomycin. These are different from many of their antibiotic
cousins, as neither are absorbed from the intestines. It can take several
weeks of treatment to get rid of SIBO, since there are generally other
underlying factors in the gut that also need to be addressed for successful treatment.

Alternatively, several herbal protocols are as effective as or more
effective than antibiotic therapy. I prefer using Candibactin-AR and
Candibactin-BR (made by Metagenics), which is an essential-oil product, plus a berberine with coptis complex. This powerful herbal combination has been shown in one study to be more effective than
rifaximin at eradicating SIBO.[10] Although this study has been criti-
cized, since the amount of rifaximin used was lower than is typically
used to treat SIBO, the findings still show that herbs work in treating
SIBO. The same study found that another similar herbal combination
of Dysbiocide and FC-Cidal (made by Biotics Research) was also effective at treating SIBO. Talk with your naturopathic physician or
functional medicine doctor if you want to start herbal therapy to treat
SIBO or to get guidance on what dose is best for you.

MADISON'S STORY

Madison is an avid outdoors person who loves horseback riding
and taking trail rides through the countrysides of Connecticut. A
few years ago, she became persistently fatigued and developed
digestive problems. Several different specialists put Madison on
numerous medications for IBS, reflux, and bloating. By the time
I met her, she was also having joint pain in her hips, night sweats,
swelling in her legs, and numbness in her feet. Her doctor had
run a standard Lyme antibody test through a local lab, which was
negative, so she was told she couldn't possibly have Lyme disease.

But her symptoms seemed to fit Lyme disease, so I ran a more comprehensive test with a different lab, which came back positive for both Lyme disease and *Babesia*. I started her on herbs, an alkaline diet, and some homeopathic remedies, which relieved her symptoms tremendously.

After a few months of treatment, 90 percent of her symptoms went away, except for numbness in her feet and some lingering digestive symptoms—gas and bloating after eating. A breath test for SIBO came back positive. After six weeks of SIBO treatment, her numbness almost completely disappeared. Now more than a year since she was treated for SIBO, she has not experienced any further neuropathy or digestive problems.

Mast Cell Activation Syndrome

Some of my patients with Lyme disease tell me they feel allergic all of the time, no matter what time of day or year. While allergic reactions involve many different cells and chemicals, mast cells are one of the key players. Mast cells play an important protective role against infection and defend us from foreign microbes. They are also involved in wound healing, growth of new blood vessels, improving immune tolerance, and maintaining the integrity of the blood-brain barrier.

Mast cells also produce many common allergic symptoms when they release their contents into the bloodstream. Existing throughout the body, mast cells are present in high concentrations in your skin and mucous membranes. An allergic response activates these cells. When the cell wall breaks apart, mast cells release histamine, which causes a runny nose, itchy eyes, scratchy throat, hives, or more serious symptoms like swelling of your lips or tongue or even difficulty breathing.

Mast cells also release other chemicals, including some that increase inflammation in the body and others that attract other immune cells to the site of infection. In most cases, mast cell activation is a relatively short process that goes away shortly after the exposure occurs. For example, someone with tree pollen allergy will feel better when the pollen count drops and there is no more irritation to the immune system. However, when this process doesn't shut off the way it should, it leaves you feeling hypersensitive and reactive to everything. Symptoms of mast cell activation include the following:

- Abdominal pain, with intestinal cramping, diarrhea, gas, bloating, or constipation
- Chest pain
- Burning sensation in the mouth
- Mouth ulcers
- Persistent cough
- Shortness of breath
- Runny nose
- Asthma-like symptoms or sinus congestion
- Chronic swollen eyes or lymph nodes
- Fast heart rate
- Abnormally high or low blood pressure
- Dizziness
- Fainting
- Flushed skin
- Hives or itchy skin
- Headaches
- Neuropathy
- Poor concentration or memory
- Sleeplessness

- Ringing in the ears
- Fatigue
- Fever or arthritis

If any of these symptoms sounds familiar to you, then you may have mast cell activation syndrome (MCAS). Allergies are the most common cause of MCAS, but studies show that Lyme disease can stimulate mast cells, causing them to release histamine and all of their other contents that trigger allergy-like symptoms.[11] The persistent spirochete in your body constantly provokes your immune system and you feel allergic all day long. The symptoms can also be heightened in Lyme. I have seen patients with Lyme disease with severe gastrointestinal problems, chronic sinus or lung congestion, and extremely sensitive skin due to MCAS.

Unfortunately, there is no good test for MCAS. The diagnosis is based primarily on your symptoms. Someone with MCAS will show elevated measures of these mast cell contents in a blood test:[12]

- *N*-methyl histamine
- Tryptase
- Heparin
- Prostaglandin D2
- Chromogranin A

I have run these tests on people with Lyme disease and occasionally they come back positive, confirming my diagnosis of MCAS. Other tests, like bone marrow biopsy, colonoscopy, or endoscopy with biopsies can look for mast cells in the tissue, but these are invasive and not commonly performed.

The treatment of MCAS entails blocking the effect of histamine.

One of the best nutrients for this is quercetin, a bioflavonoid found in several foods, with the highest amounts found in onions. Quercetin can stabilize the cell wall of mast cells so they don't release their contents when stimulated. You probably couldn't eat enough onions to treat mast cell activation syndrome (at least not without offending your friends and family), so taking it as a nutritional supplement is best. Take 500 to 1,000 milligrams twice a day before meals to keep mast cells under control. Quercetin has been shown to be more effective than some prescription medications in preventing mast cells from breaking apart.[13]

The first-line medical treatment of MCAS is over-the-counter antihistamines, such as diphenhydramine (Benadryl), cetirizine (Zyrtec), loratadine (Claritin), or fexofenadine (Allegra) to block the action of histamine.[14] If these do not work for you, talk with your doctor about using prescription antihistamines.

Antihistamines can make you feel tired, so using mast cell stabilizers may be better suited for you, with fewer side effects. They also require a doctor's prescription. Cromolyn sodium, one of the most commonly used,[15] was discovered in 1965 in an ancient Egyptian herb called khella (*Ammi visnaga*) by Dr. Roger Altounyan, who was using it to treat his own asthma. He had taken one of the ingredients in the plant and slightly altered it to make it less toxic. Commercial preparations of cromolyn sodium can be squirted up your nose (NasalCrom), inhaled (Intal), or taken orally (Gastrocrom). The nasal version is available over the counter, while the oral and inhaled versions are by prescription only. The nasal spray is used to treat hay fever, the inhaled version is for treating asthma, and the oral preparation is for preventing food allergies and MCAS. You can also have a compounding pharmacy make capsules of pure cromolyn sodium if you are sensitive to preservatives, which are found in Gastrocrom. Take 100 milligrams of cromolyn sodium ten minutes before each meal to get the most benefit. Cromolyn sodium is expensive in the United States, so try quercetin and antihistamines first. Ketotifen works similarly to cromolyn sodium and is used widely in Europe but is available in the United States only through compounding pharmacies.

Antihistamines can work quickly but only block the effect of histamine. Because mast cells release other chemicals into your blood besides histamine, you may need to use a mast cell stabilizer at the same time to get the best results. I have used combinations of these medications and nutrients and find that they work well together in controlling symptoms with minimal to no side effects.

POTS: When Your Nervous System Breaks Down

Have you ever had trouble standing up or felt dizzy or light-headed when you get up from a chair or bed? Have you ever fainted while doing just a minimal amount of exercise or work? Do you notice your heart is constantly pounding and feels fast? Have you had difficulty regulating your body temperature and find that you go from hot to cold regardless of the weather? If so, you may have postural orthostatic tachycardia syndrome (POTS).

POTS is caused by an imbalance in your nervous system that affects normal body functions, such as heart rate, breathing, perspiration, or blood flow. People with POTS may also experience the following:

- Headaches
- Nausea
- Purple hands or feet
- Anxiety

- Chest pain
- Muscle weakness
- Fatigue
- Vision changes
- Poor focus or memory

Nature designed your nervous system to adapt as your body changes position in order to maintain healthy blood flow to your whole body. When you stand up, gravity wants to pull your blood down toward your feet, so your blood vessels constrict and your heart rate speeds up a little to keep blood moving into your brain. When you have POTS, your autonomic nervous system (part of your nervous system that controls normal body functions without any conscious effort on your part, like breathing and heart rate) becomes sluggish. You feel like you want to pass out when your body is upright. This can obviously become a big problem, since people spend most of their day either sitting or standing. The inability to regulate your blood flow interferes with simple daily activities and can even become debilitating.

Several factors can lead to POTS, including trauma, surgery, chemotherapy, and infection. Lyme disease is another possible cause of POTS. Even people with chronic Lyme disease who have previously been treated with antibiotics have developed POTS.[16] Although doctors don't know what exactly causes POTS, it can be treated.

If you think you have POTS, please work with your doctor. Diagnosis is simple: measuring your blood pressure while you are lying down and then at two, five, and ten minutes after standing. If your heart rate increases by more than 30 to 40 beats per minute (bpm) after standing or goes over 120 bpm and your blood pressure drops, then you likely have POTS.

To get the best results, the treatment of POTS often involves multiple therapies. To begin with, make sure you are well hydrated and get plenty of electrolytes, such as sodium or potassium. Adding salt to your diet and eating small, frequent meals may also work to control POTS. Doing some sort of exercise can improve symptoms of POTS. If you do not exercise at all, then you may make this condition worse.[17] Several medications can also be used to treat POTS.[18] Talk with your doctor about which treatments may be best for you.

What If I Relapse?

I remember the first time I started to get symptoms of Lyme again, months after I was initially treated. I recall the feeling of panic and then denial. This couldn't possibly be Lyme again, could it? Of course not. It was the dead of winter in Connecticut and freezing outside. No ticks can survive when it's that cold, right? There is no way I got bit . . . *again*? All of these thoughts kept running through my head. I kept waiting for the symptoms to just go away. Maybe I was just stressed out and needed more sleep. Perhaps I wasn't eating as well as I should have been. But after several weeks passed and the symptoms started to worsen, it finally hit me. I was having a relapse.

My story is very common among people who have Lyme. You get to a point of feeling better or even completely symptom-free. Then you start to feel bad again. You go over in your mind, "What did I do?" You start to question everything you did prior to the flare-up. "Did I eat the wrong thing?" "Did I get another tick bite?" "Am I not sleeping enough?" "Am I not taking care of myself enough?" Maybe there was something that triggered your symptoms, but usually it's not obvious. Of course it's a good idea to take inventory of your life and note anything that may have affected your immune system or overall health. But if you begin to feel unwell again, don't delay treatment. It's easy to ignore the early signs of a relapse when you're busy or preoccupied with life.

If you restart treatment early in your flare, you can prevent things from getting out of control and keep yourself from feeling much worse. Go back through the program. Be diligent about taking care of yourself. Enact your treatment plan right away and go see your health-care provider if needed. Start with the things that worked for you before. If you find that the treatments aren't working as well as before, then you need to do something different. It may mean using a different combination of herbs, making additional diet changes, getting more sleep, taking new supplements, or seeing your doctor for a physician-guided treatment. Don't panic. Breathe. The good news is that your body is an amazing machine with a capacity to heal. I know how discouraging it can feel to relapse, but you got well before. You can do it again.

Epilogue

I didn't ask for Lyme disease and neither did you. It came into your life surreptitiously and changed you. It has disrupted your daily activities, forced you to do things you had never planned on doing, and changed you physically, mentally, and emotionally. It has taken a toll on your personal relationships, work, and school. This uninvited guest has been the party crasher we are all too happy to see leave. But it has left a mess and now we have to work to clean that mess up.

Getting through Lyme disease and the immune issues it creates is a process. You started taking steps to address these issues by reading this book and becoming proactive about your own health. The silver lining is that Lyme disease has fostered an inner strength that you may not have known you had. You are stronger than you might feel. And you are not alone. We are a worldwide brotherhood and sisterhood that have all been dealt the same card. Don't be afraid to reach out to others who have already been down this road. There is strength in numbers. We are a mighty network of information and support.

You are a Lyme warrior, armed with knowledge and determination to get well. There will be many battles to fight, but with each victory, you are one step closer to recovering and getting your life back. Find the right practitioners, people who are invested in your well-being, and make them part of your health team. Surround yourself with people who make you laugh, lift you up, and support you. There is a light at the end of this tunnel. You are on your way to restoring your body and mind to health and wellness.

Recipes

I am a simple cook at best, so I wanted to find recipes that were easy to prepare and tasted good. I worked with a nutritionist friend of mine to help develop these recipes, following the guidelines of the Immune-Boosting Diet. What I love about these recipes is that most of them can be prepared in under thirty minutes, so it does not take a lot of time to make nutritious, healthy food for you and your family.

My diet prior to transitioning to the Immune-Boosting Diet was heavy in meat. (I grew up in Southern California but was born in Indiana, so meat and potatoes were main staples of my diet as a kid.) The Immune-Boosting Diet is mostly vegetarian, so it took me a while to get into the habit of eating this new way. But once I did, I felt the difference within just a few weeks. I hope that you will have a similar experience.

The goal here isn't to eat the same recipe over and over, but to find a variety of foods that give you the full complement of nutrients your body needs to get well and maintain an alkaline pH. As I mentioned in Chapter 4, some of the foods (particularly meats and eggs) should be consumed no more than five times per week, so keep that in mind as you follow the diet plan. If you are struggling to implement the diet plan, please work with a local nutritionist or contact one of our nutritionists to help guide you on making this diet transition successful.

BREAKFAST

Morning Boost Smoothie

. . . .

MAKES 1 SERVING

My favorite green drink is so easy to make. You can get these ingredients all year round, and enjoy it all year long. Add a little extra avocado if your like your smoothie a bit thicker.

1½ to 2 cups filtered water

¼ organic avocado

½ green apple, peeled and chopped

1 tablespoon fresh organic lime juice

1 cup chopped organic rainbow Swiss chard leaves

Place all of the ingredients into a Vitamix or other heavy-duty blender and blend until smooth. If the consistency is too thick, gradually add water and blend until you reach the desired texture.

Warm Buckwheat Bowl

· ·

MAKES 4 SERVINGS

If you enjoy oatmeal as much as I do, this is an ideal alternative for a hearty breakfast. I like blueberries in mine, but fresh mango, pomegranate seeds, or raspberries can be substituted to add more variety to the dish.

¾ cup almond-coconut milk (I like Califia Farms)

1 cup filtered water

1 cup organic buckwheat groats

1 tablespoon coconut oil

⅛ teaspoon sea salt

1 teaspoon vanilla extract

1 teaspoon lo-han sweetener

1 tablespoon organic maple syrup

1 teaspoon organic ground cinnamon

Coconut chips or unsweetened shredded coconut, for topping

Slivered almonds, for topping

Organic blueberries, for topping

If you have a rice cooker, I suggest using it for this. It makes life so much easier. You can set it to the white rice setting (if you have digital) and just the normal setting if your rice cooker is not digital.

Place the milk, water, buckwheat, coconut oil, salt, vanilla, lo-han, maple syrup, and cinnamon into the rice cooker and cook according to the instructions. Once done, remove from the cooker and stir. Scoop

½ cup of the porridge into a small bowl and top with the coconut, almonds, and blueberries. Serve immediately.

To cook this on the stovetop, heat a medium saucepan over medium heat. Add the milk, water, buckwheat, coconut oil and salt. Cook for 5 to 7 minutes, then cover and simmer over low heat for 15 minutes. Remove the lid and add the vanilla, lo-han, maple syrup, and cinnamon. Cover and continue to cook over low for an additional 4 to 5 minutes. Remove from the heat, remove the lid, and allow to cool for 5 minutes. Scoop ½ cup of the porridge into a small bowl and top with the coconuts, almonds, and blueberries. Serve immediately.

Simple Detox Smoothie

MAKES 1 SERVING

This is my go-to breakfast when I'm pressed for time or traveling and want a nutrient-packed shake. I prefer it blended, but you can also put it in a shaker and mix it by hand. It works equally well as a meal substitute or a quick snack. Add more water if you like a thinner consistency.

1 scoop vanilla Ingels Detox Support Plus powder

½ cup filtered water

1 cup unsweetened almond-coconut milk

½ cup frozen organic berries

1 cup ice

1 teaspoon flaxseed or flax meal

1 tablespoon hempseed

Place all of the ingredients into a Vitamix or other heavy-duty blender and blend until smooth. If the consistency is too thick, gradually add water and blend until you reach the desired texture.

Delightful Detox Smoothie Bowl

MAKES 2 SERVINGS

Spending time in California, I've noticed the popularity of the acai bowl—filled with fresh fruit, granola, and frozen, blended acai fruit. I love it so much, I created a healthier version of it with added greens, nuts, and seeds for more protein and other nutrients. This makes a fun, tasty breakfast that you'll really enjoy.

For smoothie bowl:

1 cup packed organic baby kale leaves, washed

1 teaspoon organic spirulina powder

1 cup Califia Farms almond-coconut milk, carrageenan-free

½ organic avocado

½ teaspoon lo-han sweetener or stevia, to taste

1 scoop vanilla Ingels Detox Support Plus or Mediclear Plus powder (Thorne Research)

1½ cups ice

1 medium organic banana

8 fresh or frozen organic strawberries

For topping:

   2 organic strawberries, sliced

   ¼ cup organic raspberries

   1 tablespoon raw organic chia seeds

   1 tablespoon raw organic slivered almonds

   1 tablespoon raw organic sunflower seeds

   2 tablespoons unsweetened coconut chips

Place all of the smoothie bowl ingredients into a Vitamix or other heavy-duty blender and blend on high for 2 minutes. Pour into a medium bowl and top with the topping ingredients. Serve.

Vanilla-Almond Immune Shake

. . . .

MAKES 1 SERVING

   2 scoops vanilla Ingels Detox Support Plus powder or Mediclear Plus
      powder (Thorne Research)

   2 cups ice

   6 ounces filtered water

   4 ounces coconut-almond milk, carrageenan-free

   1 small organic banana

   1 teaspoon organic almond extract

   ¼ teaspoon lo-han sweetener

   1 teaspoon organic flax oil

   1 tablespoon organic almond butter

   ¼ cup organic pomegranate seeds, for topping

Place the vanilla powder, ice, water, milk, banana, almond extract, lo-han, and flax oil in a Vitamix or other heavy-duty blender. Pulse on high for 20 seconds, then add the almond butter and blend on high for 1 to 2 minutes. Pour into a glass and top with the pomegranate seeds. Serve and enjoy.

LUNCH

Chickpea, Avocado, and Cherry Tomato Salad

· ·

MAKES 3 TO 4 SERVINGS

For salad:

16 ounces cooked organic chickpeas

1 organic red onion, diced

1 cup organic cherry tomatoes, chopped

1 organic avocado, diced into 1-inch pieces

2 teaspoons dried organic oregano

⅓ cup finely chopped fresh organic flat-leaf parsley

1 organic English cucumber, diced

For dressing:

2 tablespoons fresh organic lemon juice

¼ cup extra-virgin olive oil

2 cloves organic garlic, minced

Cracked black pepper, to taste

Sea salt, to taste

In a medium bowl, combine the chickpeas, onion, tomatoes, and avocado and stir. Next, sprinkle the oregano and parsley over the mixture.

In a small bowl, combine the dressing ingredients and whisk until creamy. Pour the dressing over the chickpea mixture, toss, and stir to coat evenly. Add more salt if needed. Serve.

Detox Salad

MAKES 4 TO 5 SERVINGS

For salad:

1 cup shredded organic carrots

2 organic beets, shredded or diced

½ organic red onion, diced

½ cup organic purple cabbage, shredded

2 cups organic dandelion greens, roughly chopped

2 cups organic mustard greens, roughly chopped

¼ cup organic chopped parsley

¼ cup organic chopped cilantro

2 tablespoons raw sunflower seeds

2 tablespoons raw pumpkin seeds

For dressing:

½ cup extra-virgin olive oil

¼ cup coconut vinegar

1 clove organic garlic, minced

¼ teaspoon sea salt

Cracked black pepper, to taste

In a large bowl, combine the salad ingredients.

In a small bowl, whisk together the dressing ingredients until creamy. Drizzle over the salad and toss to incorporate evenly. Sprinkle with additional sea salt and pepper, if desired. Serve.

Crunchy Marinated Kale Salad

MAKES 4 SERVINGS

Kale is packed with several minerals, especially calcium and iron. I try to eat kale at least three times per week. If you find kale too bitter for your taste, you can substitute Swiss chard, which has a milder flavor. Add a little extra avocado if you want to get more healthy fat in your diet.

For salad:

5 cups packed organic kale leaves, stems removed

2 ounces organic cashew nuts, chopped

¼ cup toasted sesame seeds

½ cup raw sunflower seeds

1 cup shredded organic carrots

1 organic avocado, diced

½ medium red onion, diced

For dressing:

¼ cup extra-virgin olive oil

2 tablespoons coconut vinegar

1 teaspoon fresh organic lemon juice

1 tablespoon coconut aminos

¼ teaspoon sea salt, or more to taste

Cracked black pepper, to taste

Wash and dry the kale leaves and chop them into 2-inch pieces. In a large bowl combine the salad ingredients. In a small bowl, whisk together the dressing ingredients until creamy. Pour the dressing over the salad and massage the dressing into the kale with gloved hands to ensure an even coating of dressing on everything. Cover and refrigerate for 1 hour. Remove from the refrigerator and serve.

Spicy Cabbage Slaw

MAKES APPROXIMATELY 7 SERVINGS

This twist on coleslaw is perfect if you like more spicy food. By adding or subtracting cayenne pepper, you can adjust this recipe to your preferences. Cayenne pepper can help improve your circulation, so if you can tolerate more, it will help get your blood moving.

For slaw:

½ head organic green cabbage, shredded

½ head organic purple cabbage, shredded

1 cup shredded organic carrots

½ organic red onion, thinly sliced

⅓ cup thinly sliced scallions

For dressing:

> 3 tablespoons coconut vinegar
>
> 2 tablespoons organic coconut nectar
>
> ½ teaspoon organic garlic powder
>
> 1 teaspoon sea salt
>
> ⅓ cup extra virgin olive oil
>
> ⅛ teaspoon organic cayenne pepper

In a large bowl, combine the salad ingredients. In a medium bowl, whisk together the dressing ingredients until creamy. Pour the dressing over the cabbage mixture and toss thoroughly to coat. Cover and refrigerate for 1 hour. Remove from the refrigerator and serve.

Arugula, Beet, and Super-Seed Salad

. . . .

MAKES 1 TO 2 SERVINGS

Beets are a great source of vitamin C, B vitamins, folate, potassium, and fiber. The arugula and seeds round the plate out with a crunchy quality. Goes well with any entrée.

For salad:

> 2½ cups packed organic arugula
>
> 2 small organic beets, chopped into 1-inch pieces
>
> 8 organic Sunfood brand black Peruvian olives
>
> 1 tablespoon organic hempseed

1 tablespoon organic sunflower seeds

1 tablespoon organic raw pumpkin seeds

For dressing:

2 teaspoons minced organic garlic

2 tablespoons organic flax oil

1 tablespoon plus 1 teaspoon coconut vinegar

2 teaspoons kimchi liquid (just the liquid from the kimchi bottle)

1 tablespoon pumpkin seed oil

¼ teaspoon coconut aminos

½ teaspoon coconut nectar

½ teaspoon dried organic oregano

⅛ teaspoon sea salt

Cracked black pepper, to taste

Arrange the arugula on a medium plate. Place the beets, olives, and hempseed on top.

In a small bowl, combine the dressing ingredients and whisk until smooth, 1 to 2 minutes.

Pour the dressing over the salad and toss to incorporate the dressing evenly. Serve.

Chicken, Greens, and Quinoa Salad

MAKES 4 SERVINGS

1 pound organic chicken breast (pasture-raised is best)

1 teaspoon sea salt

8 cups mixed greens such as mesclun or baby arugula

1 cup cooked organic quinoa

Extra-virgin olive oil, to taste

Juice of 3 to 4 organic lemons

Cracked black pepper, to taste

Boil water in a medium stockpot. Add the chicken and salt and cook until tender, 12 to 15 minutes. Remove from the heat, remove the chicken from the pot, slice it, and place it in a medium bowl. Divide the greens among 4 dinner plates and sprinkle ¼ cup cooked quinoa over each plate. Add 4 ounces chicken on top of each plate, in the center. Drizzle with olive oil and fresh lemon juice, and sprinkle with cracked pepper. Serve.

Healthy Gut Kimchi Roll

MAKES 12 ROLLS

12 to 14 organic Swiss chard leaves (6 to 7 inches wide and 8 to 9

inches long)

3 tablespoons coconut aminos

1½ cups cooked quinoa

1½ cups kimchi

½ cup sauerkraut

1½ organic avocados

Wash the Swiss chard leaves thoroughly and inspect them for any tears. Do not use torn leaves. Cut off the thick stem at the end of each leaf.

Fill a large pot with 1 inch of warm water and place a bamboo steamer in the pot. Arrange the leaves in the steamer in opposite directions to cover the bottom of the steamer completely.

Place the lid on the pot and steam over medium-high heat for 10 to 13 minutes. After 8 minutes, check the leaves to see if they have softened. Use a fork to poke into the thickest part of the leaf and stem. If it is difficult to push the fork through, return the leaves to the steamer and cook for another 5 minutes. If is the leaves are soft, but not soggy, then they are ready.

Remove from the heat. Remove the lid and wait for the steam to dissipate. Pull out the leaves gently with tongs and place them on a plate. Run the plate with the leaves under cold water for 1 to 2 minutes or until the leaves have cooled completely.

Drain the leaves and pat each leaf dry with an unbleached paper towel or cloth.

Assemble the filling ingredients in separate bowls.

Mix the coconut aminos into the cooked quinoa. Set aside.

Mix the kimchi with the sauerkraut and set aside.

Cut the avocado in half and remove the pit. Take each half and make slices lengthwise with a knife. You should be able to get 7 to 8 slices from each half.

Next, placing one leaf at a time on a plate, add 1 tablespoon quinoa, then the kimchi mixture, then 2 avocado slices on top. It should be all in a neat small pile in the middle of the leaf. Make sure you have about 2 inches of leaf on each side of the pile. Take the side of the leaf closest to you and roll it up to cover the pile. Take the two opposite ends of the leaf and fold over toward the middle of the pile. Then roll the leaf toward the open end (think of folding a burrito). Turn the roll over on the opposite side and place it on a plate. These can be a little messy, but they are well worth it.

Hijiki Seaweed Salad

MAKES 4 SERVINGS

4 ounces hijiki seaweed, soaked for 30 minutes in water and drained
   thoroughly

¼ cup organic shredded carrots

1 tablespoon organic flax oil

2 tablespoons plus 1 teaspoon coconut vinegar

2 teaspoons grated fresh organic ginger

⅓ cup coconut aminos

4 tablespoons sesame seeds, raw or dry-toasted

Place the drained seaweed and the carrots in a medium bowl and set aside. In a small bowl, whisk together the flax oil, vinegar, ginger, and coconut aminos until the mixture is almost creamy and does not separate. Pour the dressing onto the seaweed and toss to coat thoroughly. Sprinkle with the sesame seeds and serve.

SOUPS AND BROTHS

Ingels's Lentil Soup

MAKES 4 SERVINGS

4 tablespoons extra-virgin olive oil

2 cloves organic garlic, minced

1 medium organic yellow onion, diced

2 cups vegetable broth

3 cups filtered water

¾ cup dry red lentils

1 organic celery stalk, finely chopped

1 large organic carrot, finely chopped

2 teaspoons sea salt

2 teaspoons organic ground coriander

1 teaspoon organic ground cumin

¼ teaspoon cracked black pepper

2 tablespoons fresh organic lemon juice

In a large stockpot over medium-high heat, heat 2 tablespoons of the olive oil, then add the garlic and onion and sauté for 5 to 6 minutes. Add the broth, water, lentils, celery, carrot, salt, coriander, cumin, and pepper. Reduce the heat to medium-low, cover, and simmer for 20 to 25 minutes. Add more salt if necessary and stir. Add the lemon juice and the remaining 2 tablespoons olive oil. Remove from the heat and allow to cool for 5 minutes before serving.

Quick Immune-Soothing Bone Broth

. . . .

MAKES 5 SERVINGS

2 tablespoons extra-virgin organic coconut oil

1 cup finely chopped organic leeks

2 cloves organic garlic, minced

1 (32-oz.) carton Pacific brand unsalted bone stock

2 teaspoons Frontier brand organic adobo

1 teaspoon Frontier brand muchi curry powder

1 teaspoon fresh organic lime juice

½ teaspoon grated fresh organic ginger

½ cup organic full-fat coconut milk

3 tablespoons organic coconut vinegar

1½ tablespoons coconut aminos

In a cast-iron stockpot, over medium-high heat, combine the coconut oil, leeks, and garlic and sauté for 4 minutes, stirring occasionally. Add the bone stock, adobo, curry powder, lime juice, ginger, coconut milk, coconut vinegar, and coconut aminos and stir. Reduce the heat to medium-low and simmer for 7 minutes. Remove from the heat and allow to cool for five minutes. Pour into bowls and serve.

Simple Vegetable Broth

. . . .

MAKES APPROXIMATELY 10 CUPS

3 tablespoons avocado oil

3 organic yellow onions, roughly chopped

4 cloves organic garlic, smashed

2 organic leeks, roughly chopped

3 quarts filtered water

3 organic carrots, roughly chopped

4 organic thyme sprigs

3 organic celery stalks, roughly chopped

1 teaspoon organic ground coriander

1 tablespoon fresh organic lemon juice

2 teaspoons sea salt

Cracked black pepper, to taste

In a large stockpot over medium-high heat, combine the avocado oil, onions, garlic, and leeks and sauté for 7 minutes, stirring occasionally. Add the remaining ingredients, bring to a boil, then cover and reduce the heat to medium-low and simmer for 1 hour.

Remove from the heat. Pour the mixture through a large strainer into a large bowl.

You can freeze this broth for 2 months or bottle it in glass jars once it has cooled. It can be refrigerated for up to 5 days.

Carrot, Ginger, and Squash Soup

MAKES 6 TO 7 SERVINGS

3 tablespoons organic coconut oil

2 yellow onions, diced

2 cloves organic garlic, minced

2 tablespoons grated fresh ginger

2 quarts filtered water

½ pound yellow squash, cut into 1-inch slices

5 organic carrots, cut into ½-inch slices

3 tablespoons extra-virgin olive oil

2 teaspoons sea salt

Cracked black pepper, to taste

In a large stockpot over medium heat, combine 1 tablespoon of the coconut oil with the onions and garlic and sauté for 4 to 5 minutes. Add the remaining ingredients, reduce the heat to medium, and cover and simmer for 20 to 25 minutes or until the vegetables are soft. Remove from the heat. Using an immersion blender, purée until completely smooth. Add more salt and pepper if needed. Serve in small bowls.

Celeriac and Fennel Soup

. . . .

MAKES 5 SERVINGS

If you have never had celeriac (celery root) before, you are in for a treat. This delicious soup is robust with flavor and has a wonderful, creamy texture. The fennel adds a subtle savory flavor. If it seems too strong for you, just use one fennel bulb the next time you make it. This is a nice warming soup for those cold, damp days.

2 organic celery root bulbs

2 organic fennel bulbs

1 large yellow onion

3 cloves organic garlic, minced

¼ cup extra-virgin olive oil

¼ cup full-fat coconut milk (Natural Value or Native Forest)

10 cups filtered water

4 tablespoons fresh lemon juice

1 tablespoon sea salt

Cracked black pepper, to taste

Wash and peel the celery root bulbs and chop them into 2-inch pieces. Wash the fennel bulbs and chop them into 2-inch pieces. Chop the onion into 2-inch pieces as well.

In a large stockpot over medium-high heat, combine all of the ingredients. Bring to a boil, cover, and reduce heat. Simmer for 20 to 25 minutes or until the vegetables are very tender and soft. Remove from the heat and allow to cool for 15 minutes. Purée the soup in 2 batches in a blender.

Serve immediately.

BREADS AND CRACKERS

Cassava and Multi-Seed Flatbread

MAKES 4 FLATBREADS

1 cup cassava flour

½ teaspoon sea salt

2 tablespoons raw sunflower seeds

2 tablespoons raw pumpkin seeds

1 tablespoon flaxseed

¾ cup warm water

2 tablespoons olive or avocado oil

⅛ teaspoon lo-han sweetener or 1 teaspoon coconut nectar

Safflower oil (for greasing the pan)

Preheat the oven to 450°F. Mix together the flour, salt, and seeds. Add the warm water and knead the dough, incorporating all flour and seeds until smooth. If the dough is still dry, add 2 tablespoons water at a time until the consistency is doughlike but not too wet. Add the olive oil and lo-han sweetener or coconut nectar and work it into the dough.

Divide the dough into 4 even-size balls and roll each ball between two pieces of unbleached parchment paper. With your hand or a rolling pin, roll out the dough to about ½-inch thick. Lightly grease the baking pan with safflower oil. Transfer the rolled-out dough to a baking pan.

Bake for 8 to 9 minutes, then remove from the oven, flip the flatbread over, and bake for another 5 to 6 minutes, until it is slightly soft in the middle and the bubbles that have formed around the middle and edges are light golden brown.

Super-Seed Crackers

SERVINGS VARY DEPENDING ON HOW YOU CUT THEM

2 tablespoons organic flax seeds

2 tablespoons organic chia seeds

1 teaspoon organic onion powder

½ cup raw organic sunflower seeds

½ cup raw organic pumpkin seeds

4 ounces organic almond flour

Hot filtered water

1 teaspoon sea salt

1 teaspoon organic garlic powder

Preheat the oven to 325°F. In a small bowl, combine the seeds and the almond flour. Pour 1½ cups hot water over the seed mixture and stir. Allow to sit for about 20 minutes. If the mixture is too dry and breaking up after 20 minutes, add ½ cup hot water and mix. The consistency should be somewhat wet and doughlike. If you need to add more water, do so. Line a cookie sheet with unbleached parchment paper.

Scoop the seed mixture onto the cookie sheet and flatten with a rolling pin. Place another sheet of parchment paper on top of the dough. With the rolling pin, flatten the dough to about 3 millimeters thick. Next, with a dull knife or dough cutter, score the dough into cracker-size pieces. Bake for 30 minutes. Remove from the oven, flip the crackers, and bake for another 20 to 30 minutes, until golden and crispy. Times can vary depending on the weather and the type of oven, so it's important to watch them while they are baking.

Once they are done, remove them from the oven, allow to cool, then break the crackers apart. Serve plain or with the sauce or dip of your choice.

Brussels Sprout Chips

MAKES 2 SERVINGS

These chips are a fantastic substitute for potato or corn chips. Brussels sprouts are filled with many vitamins and minerals. I like to sauté or roast them. They pair well with my Pomegranate and Avocado Salsa (page 302) for a delicious snack.

½ pound organic Brussels sprouts

2 tablespoons extra-virgin olive oil

½ to 1 teaspoon sea salt

¼ teaspoon organic garlic powder

Preheat the oven to 350°F. Remove the leaves from the sprouts, peeling away layers carefully so as not to tear them. You may need to trim the stem if the leaves are not coming off. This will loosen up the leaves and make it easier to pick them off. Place the leaves on a baking sheet and spray or drizzle them with olive oil and sprinkle with sea salt and garlic. Toss to coat evenly and spread them in a single layer across a baking sheet. Bake for 7 minutes, then remove from the oven, toss to prevent burning, and bake for another 4 to 5 minutes, until crispy and golden brown. Serve immediately.

DRESSINGS AND SAUCES

Citrus Green Tahini Dressing

This is one of my favorite salad dressings. I like to make a bigger batch to keep in the refrigerator for other meals. Just double the recipe if you want to enjoy it throughout your week on salads, with fresh vegetables, or over some lightly sautéed greens.

2 cloves organic garlic, smashed

1 teaspoon sea salt

½ cup chopped fresh organic cilantro

1 tablespoon extra-virgin olive oil

½ cup tahini

½ teaspoon organic ground coriander

2 tablespoons fresh organic lemon juice

¼ cup filtered water (more if you like it thinner)

In a food processor or Vitamix, combine the garlic, salt, and cilantro and blend for 1 minute. Add the olive oil, tahini, coriander, and lemon juice. Continue processing and drizzle the water in slowly, until the consistency reaches a yogurtlike texture. Add salt to taste and process for 15 more seconds. Transfer to a jar and cover. Can be stored in the refrigerator for up to 4 days.

Egg-Free Mayo

. . . .

MAKES 2 CUPS

⅓ cup aquafaba (the liquid that is left over from a can/package of
   garbanzo beans)

⅛ teaspoon cream of tartar

⅛ teaspoon onion powder

⅛ teaspoon garlic powder

½ teaspoon pink Himalayan sea salt

Scant ⅛ teaspoon ground turmeric

⅛ teaspoon organic, ground mustard

2 teaspoons of liquid from kimchi, sauerkraut, or fermented pickles

2 teaspoons fresh lemon juice

2 teaspoons raw coconut nectar or ⅛ teaspoon lo-han

2 teaspoons coconut vinegar or apple cider vinegar

½ teaspoon plus ¼ teaspoon psyllium husk powder

¾ cup avocado oil

¼ cup olive oil

Combine the aquafaba and cream of tartar in a stainless steel bowl. Using a hand mixer, mix on high for about 1 minute. Add the onion powder, garlic powder, salt, turmeric, and ground mustard and mix to combine Add in the liquid from the kimchi, the lemon juice, coconut nectar, and coconut vinegar and mix for 1 minute or until soft peaks form. The mixture should resemble a fluffy meringue. Mix in the psyllium husk powder.

Combine the oils in a measuring cup, and slowly drizzle the oil mixture into the aquafaba mixture. It will take about 4 to 5 minutes for the mixture to incorporated and becomes thick like mayonnaise. (It will be lighter and fluffier than regular mayonnaise.).

This mayo can be stored in the refrigerator, in a covered Mason jar, for up to 10 days.

Roasted Garlic Sauce and Marinade

MAKES 1 CUP

2 cloves roasted organic garlic

4 tablespoons extra-virgin olive oil

2 tablespoons fresh organic lemon juice

1 tablespoon coconut vinegar

Leaves from 2 fresh thyme sprigs

1 teaspoon dried oregano

1 tablespoon coconut aminos

½ teaspoon organic mustard powder

Place all of the ingredients into a food processor or blender and pulse for 1 to 2 minutes. Use to marinate poultry or meats, or add to vegetables before roasting.

Chunky Tomato and Garlic Salsa

. . . .

MAKES 4½ CUPS

7 medium organic tomatoes, diced

1 large organic red onion, diced

5 cloves organic garlic, minced

¼ cup chopped organic cilantro

1½ teaspoons sea salt

1 teaspoon cracked black pepper

⅓ cup extra-virgin olive oil

5 tablespoons fresh organic lime juice

Zest of one organic lime

Combine all of the ingredients in a medium glass bowl, and toss to incorporate evenly. Refrigerate until ready to serve.

Turmeric and Garlic Hummus

. . . .

MAKES APPROXIMATELY 7 SERVINGS

Hummus is one of my favorite snacks. It also happens to be nutrient-dense as well, packed with protein and healthy fats. I like to make a large batch of it and snack on it throughout the week. Grab some of your favorite fresh-cut vegetables and dip them into the hummus for a quick snack.

1 tablespoon extra-virgin olive oil

2 cloves organic garlic

2 pounds cooked chickpeas, rinsed and drained

5 tablespoons fresh organic lemon juice

⅓ cup tahini

1½ teaspoons fresh-grated turmeric or ½ teaspoon ground turmeric

1 teaspoon sea salt

Cracked black pepper, to taste

3 to 6 tablespoons filtered water

Place the olive oil and garlic in a food processor and pulse for 10-second intervals until the garlic is minced. Next, add chickpeas, lemon juice, tahini, turmeric, salt, and pepper. Process on high for 2 minutes, then stop to add 3 tablespoons water. Continue processing until smooth. If you want it a bit thinner, add water 1 tablespoon at a time until you reach the desired consistency. Continue to process for a total of 3 to 4 minutes. Serve with organic celery and carrots or vegetables of choice.

Pomegranate and Avocado Salsa

MAKES 4 SERVINGS

Raised in Southern California, I grew up eating salsa. This is a great twist on a classic salsa. The pomegranate juice gives it an entirely different flavor. I enjoy this with black bean or lentil chips, or as a topping over a piece of wild fish or chicken breast.

1 clove organic garlic, minced

1 tablespoon fresh organic lime juice

Zest of 1 organic lime

½ cup diced red onion

½ cup chopped fresh organic cilantro

⅓ cup organic pomegranate juice

1 teaspoon sea salt

Cracked black pepper, to taste

12 ounces organic pomegranate seeds

1 organic avocado, diced

In a medium bowl, combine all of the ingredients and stir to incorporate. Season to taste. Chill until ready to serve.

Spinach-Basil Pesto

MAKES 3 TO 4 SERVINGS

My version of classic pesto includes spinach to supply extra nutrients. Since I am also gluten-free and dairy-free, I like this served over zucchini noodles or rice noodles, or as a delicious topping for grilled chicken or turkey breast.

2 cups fresh organic basil

1 cup fresh organic spinach

1 cup fresh organic parsley

1 tablespoon nutritional yeast

Sea salt, to taste

Cracked black pepper, to taste

½ cup sunflower seeds

2 cloves organic garlic

3 tablespoons extra-virgin olive oil

½ cup filtered water

Place all of the ingredients into a Vitamix or other heavy-duty blender and blend on high for 2 minutes or until the mixture is completely smooth. If the consistency is too thick, gradually add water and blend until you reach the desired texture.

Arugula and Fennel Pesto

MAKES APPROXIMATELY 16 OUNCES

3 cups organic baby arugula or wild arugula

¼ cup raw organic pumpkin seeds

3 cloves organic garlic

1 organic fennel bulb, sliced thin

4 tablespoons fresh organic lemon juice

2 tablespoons nutritional yeast

2 tablespoons organic flax oil

⅓ cup extra-virgin olive oil

Sea salt and cracked black pepper, to taste

Place the arugula, seeds, garlic, fennel, lemon juice, yeast, and flax oil in a Vitamix or other heavy-duty blender and blend until smooth.

While the machine is running, drizzle the olive oil in slowly until you reach the desired consistency. Add salt and pepper, to taste. Serve with veggies, zucchini noodles, or Miracle Noodles or use as a dip for seed crackers. Pour into a glass jar, cover, and keep refrigerated.

Artichoke, Spinach, and Olive Tapenade

MAKES APPROXIMATELY 2 CUPS

I can never get enough of this tapenade. This trio of flavors goes well with many foods. While I suggest serving it with my Super-Seed Crackers (page 295) or vegetables, I like it as a stand-alone side dish as well.

> 1 clove organic garlic, minced
>
> 10 ounces organic artichokes, frozen (defrosted), or BPA-free canned artichoke hearts
>
> Sea salt, to taste
>
> ¼ cup extra-virgin olive oil
>
> 2 tablespoons avocado oil
>
> 1 tablespoon fresh organic lemon juice
>
> 8 ounces Sunfood brand black Peruvian olives
>
> ⅛ teaspoon cayenne pepper, optional

Place all of the ingredients in a Vitamix or other heavy-duty blender and pulse until the mixture becomes smooth but still remains a bit chunky.

Add salt, if necessary. Can be served with crackers or raw veggies. Store in an airtight container in the refrigerator for up to 5 days.

DINNER

Curried Turkey Breast with Okra

MAKES 4 SERVINGS

3 tablespoons organic coconut oil

1 medium organic yellow onion, diced

3 cloves organic garlic, minced

*1 pound organic turkey breast (pasture-raised is best), cut into
   4-ounce portions*

1 cup filtered water

2½ cups frozen okra (do not thaw)

1 tablespoon Frontier brand organic adobo powder

2 teaspoons Frontier brand muchi curry powder

½ teaspoon sea salt, to taste

1 tablespoon fresh organic lemon juice

In a cast-iron stockpot over medium-high heat, combine the coconut oil, onion, and garlic and sauté for 4 to 5 minutes. Add the turkey and ½ cup of the filtered water. Cook for 4 minutes, then add in the okra, adobo, curry powder, lemon juice, and salt. Stir well, add the remaining ½ cup water, cover, and simmer for another 12 minutes, or until the meat is tender and the juices run clear. Remove from the heat, allow to cool 5 minutes, and serve.

Maitake Mushroom
and Cauliflower Stir-Fry

MAKES 6 SERVINGS

3 tablespoons avocado oil

1 large red onion, diced

3 medium organic carrots, cut into ¼-inch slices

1 head organic cauliflower, processed into "rice" using a food processor

1 tablespoon grated fresh organic ginger

3 cloves organic garlic, minced

2 cups sliced shiitake mushrooms

1 cup chopped maitake mushrooms

½ teaspoon sea salt

1½ cups frozen organic peas, defrosted

4 tablespoons coconut vinegar

6 tablespoons coconut aminos

2 tablespoons Red Boat brand fish sauce

1 teaspoon fresh organic lime juice

In a large stainless-steel skillet over medium-high heat, combine the avocado oil, onion, and carrots and sauté for 4 minutes. Add the cauliflower, ginger, garlic, mushrooms, and salt and sauté for 2 minutes. Add the peas, coconut vinegar, coconut aminos, fish sauce, and lime juice and mix well, stirring to evenly incorporate all of the ingredients. Sauté for 6 to 7 minutes, stirring every 2 minutes. Remove from the heat and allow to rest for 2 to 3 minutes.

Kale, Turkey, and Butternut Squash Bowl

. . . .

MAKES 4 SERVINGS

3 tablespoons organic extra-virgin coconut oil

1½ pounds butternut squash, chopped into 2-inch pieces

1 large red onion, diced

2 cloves organic garlic, minced

½ cup filtered water

1 teaspoon sea salt

4 cups organic kale, stems removed, chopped into 2-inch pieces

2 teaspoons fresh organic thyme leaves

1 pound organic ground turkey, white or dark meat

1 tablespoon organic lemon juice

In a cast-iron stockpot over medium-high heat, combine 2 tablespoons of the coconut oil with the onion and garlic and sauté for 3 to 4 minutes. Add the butternut squash and water and ½ teaspoon of the sea salt and stir. Reduce the heat to medium, cover, and cook for 6 minutes. Remove the cover, add the kale, and stir. Add 1 teaspoon of the thyme. Cover and simmer for another 5 to 6 minutes.

While that cooks, in a separate stainless-steel skillet over medium-high heat, combine the remaining 1 tablespoon coconut oil and the ground turkey. With a wooden spoon or spatula, break up the meat into smaller pieces and cook for about 6 minutes, until no pink is visible. Add the remaining ½ teaspoon sea salt and stir. Add the lemon juice and remaining 1 teaspoon thyme and stir, and cook for 1 minute.

Remove the turkey from the skillet, add it to the butternut squash mixture, and stir to incorporate. Remove from the heat and serve.

Vegan Zucchini Lasagna

MAKES 4 TO 5 SERVINGS

This vegan variation is a delicious alternative to the classic lasagna— one of my favorite Italian foods. While there's longer prep time than in my other recipes, it is worth it. I never knew zucchini could be so flavorful until I tried this dish. You'll be surprised how good the finished meal tastes.

2 organic zucchini

8 ounces Kite Hill ricotta-style almond cheese

1½ cups chopped shiitake mushrooms

1 cup peas, fresh or defrosted from frozen

1 cup chopped organic spinach

Fresh basil, for garnish

For sauce:

2 tablespoons extra-virgin olive oil

1 red onion, diced

3 cloves organic garlic, minced

3 medium organic carrots, cut into ½-inch slices

1 large organic beet, peeled and chopped

1 cup filtered water

2 teaspoons coconut nectar or a pinch of lo-han sweetener

2 teaspoons fresh organic lemon juice

½ teaspoon sea salt

½ teaspoon dried organic basil

½ teaspoon dried organic oregano

¼ teaspoon dried organic marjoram

In a medium stockpot over medium-high heat, combine the olive oil, onion, garlic, and carrots and sauté for 10 to 12 minutes. Next, add the beet and water, cover, and simmer for 25 to 30 minutes. remove from the heat and allow to cool for 15 minutes. Transfer the mixture to a Vitamix or other heavy-duty blender and process on high. Add the coconut nectar, lemon juice, salt, basil, oregano, and marjoram and continue to blend until the mixture is completely smooth. If the consistency is too thick, gradually add water and blend until you reach the desired texture. Set aside.

To assemble:

Preheat the oven to 375°F. Slice the zucchini lengthwise with a knife into about ¼-inch slices. In a medium baking dish or oven-safe casserole dish with a lid, place the zucchini slices side by side, covering the bottom of the dish. Spread a thin layer of ricotta cheese over the zucchini slices, then sprinkle mushrooms, peas, and spinach over the cheese and spread a thin layer of sauce on top. Repeat this for the next few layers. Top with sauce, cover, and bake for 25 minutes. Remove from the oven, remove the cover, and bake for another 20 minutes. Allow to cool for 5 to 10 minutes before serving.

Citrus, Red Onion, and Coconut Chicken

MAKES 4 SERVINGS

This is one of my favorite recipes. I like the combination of the sweetness from the coconut milk and the tanginess of the lime juice. It is light and refreshing, yet still a hearty meal. Add a little extra lime juice if you like it a bit more tangy.

5 tablespoons extra-virgin olive oil

¼ cup coconut milk (Natural Value or Native Forest brand)

2 organic garlic cloves

4 tablespoons fresh organic lime juice

¼ cup filtered water

1 teaspoon sea salt

1 tablespoon chopped organic cilantro

1 tablespoon chopped organic flat-leaf parsley

1 medium red onion, diced

4 organic boneless, skinless chicken breasts, 5 ounces each
  (pasture-raised is best)

In a small bowl, combine 4 tablespoons of the olive oil with the coconut milk, garlic, lime juice, water, salt, cilantro, and parsley. Transfer the mixture to a food processor or blender and pulse or blend on high for 1 to 2 minutes. In a large sauté pan over medium heat, combine the remaining 1 tablespoon olive oil and the onion and sauté for 3 to 4 minutes. Add the mixture from the food processor. Add the chicken breasts, spoon the mixture over the chicken, cover, and cook for 7 minutes. Remove the cover, stir, flip the chicken, and cook for another 7 minutes. Add ¼ cup more water, if necessary. The chicken is ready when the internal temperature reaches 165°F. Remove from the heat and allow to cool for 5 minutes. Serve the chicken topped with spoonfuls of the pan sauce.

Anti-Inflammatory Butternut Squash Stew

MAKES 5 SERVINGS

3 tablespoons organic coconut oil

1 large red onion, diced

2 cloves organic garlic, diced

2 cups organic vegetable stock

2 tablespoons Frontier brand organic adobo

1½ tablespoons Frontier brand muchi curry powder

4 ounces organic coconut milk (Natural Value or Native Forest brand)

5 cups organic butternut squash, cut into 2-inch cubes

2 tablespoons fresh organic lime juice

Sea salt and cracked black pepper, to taste

In a large stockpot over medium heat, combine the coconut oil, onion, and garlic and sauté for 5 minutes, stirring occasionally. Add the stock, adobo, curry powder, coconut milk, and squash. Stir to incorporate the ingredients evenly, cover, and simmer for 10 minutes. Add lime juice, salt, and pepper and stir. Cover and simmer for another 3 to 5 minutes. The stew is done when the butternut squash is fork-tender and falls apart. Allow to cool for 5 minutes before serving.

SIDES

Roasted Cauliflower Rice

MAKES 4 SERVINGS

1 head organic cauliflower

3 to 4 tablespoons extra-virgin olive oil

1 teaspoon sea salt

Cracked black pepper, to taste

Preheat the oven to 400°F. In a large bowl, combine all of the ingredients and toss to coat evenly. On a large cookie sheet, spread the "rice" flat evenly across the whole sheet. Bake for 20 minutes. Remove and stir, then bake for another 10 minutes or until golden brown. Remove from the oven, allow to cool for 5 minutes, and serve.

Chipotle Avocado Mash

MAKES APPROXIMATELY 1½ CUPS

3 tablespoons fresh organic lime juice

2 ripe organic avocados, mashed with a fork

⅛ teaspoon chipotle powder

1 tablespoon extra-virgin olive oil

¼ teaspoon sea salt

¼ cup chopped fresh organic cilantro

Combine all of the ingredients in a glass bowl and stir to incorporate evenly. Serve or refrigerate immediately.

Cast-Iron Roasted Sunchokes and Burdock Root

MAKES 6 TO 7 SERVINGS

If you like artichokes, then you'll love sunchokes. Their texture is like a soft potato, but their flavor is similar to an artichoke's. Also known as Jerusalem artichokes, they grow between October and February and can be difficult to find at other times of the year.

This is a great dish to help support your liver and promote detoxification. I try to make this dish whenever sunchokes are in season.

1½ pounds burdock root, scrubbed, washed, and cut into

   ½-inch slices

1 pound sunchokes, washed and cut into ½-inch pieces

4 cloves organic garlic, minced

¼ cup olive oil or coconut oil

½ teaspoon sea salt

2 tablespoons coconut aminos

Cracked black pepper, to taste

Preheat the oven to 375°F. In a cast-iron, oven-safe pan, combine all of the ingredients and toss to coat all pieces evenly. Bake for 35 to 40 minutes or until golden brown and slightly crispy. Allow to cool for 5 minutes. Serve.

Mashed-Up Veggie Delight

MAKES 5 TO 6 SERVINGS

10 cups filtered water

½ pound organic turnips, peeled and cubed into 1-inch pieces

½ pound organic cauliflower, cut into 2-inch pieces

½ pound organic carrots, cut into 1-inch slices

1 medium organic yellow onion, chopped

1 teaspoon sea salt

Cracked black pepper, to taste

3 tablespoons organic coconut oil

In a medium stockpot, combine the water, turnips, cauliflower, carrots, and onion. Cover, bring to a boil, and cook for 15 minutes or until tender. Remove from the heat and drain. Transfer the vegetables to a food processor and add the salt, pepper, and coconut oil. Process for 2 minutes or until smooth.

Lemon-Sesame Green Beans

....

MAKES 4 SERVINGS

Green beans are one of my favorite vegetables. I love that you can find fresh or frozen organic green beans throughout the year. This easy-to-make dish is perfect when your time is limited, as it can be prepared in less than 10 minutes.

1 pound organic green beans (frozen is great, too)

4 tablespoons extra-virgin olive oil

2 tablespoons fresh organic lemon juice

1 teaspoon sea salt

3 tablespoons Eden brand Garlic Gomasio (this is a mixture of toasted sesame seeds, sea salt, and garlic)

Fill a medium stockpot with 2 to 3 inches of water. Add the green beans, cover, bring to a boil, and cook for 5 to 6 minutes. Stir twice while boiling. Remove from the heat and drain well. In a medium sauté pan, combine the olive oil and green beans and sauté over medium heat for 2 minutes. Add the lemon juice and salt and stir to incorporate. Remove from the heat. Add the Gomasio and stir again. Allow to cool for 2 to 3 minutes and serve.

Flu-Fighter Immune Fries

. . . .

MAKES 5 SERVINGS

There is nothing like homemade fries. Using sweet potatoes instead of white potatoes gives you more beta carotene, B vitamins, vitamin C, and fiber. I'm a big fan of curry, so the blend of curry powder with adobo gives these fries a unique, zesty flavor that you'll love.

2 pounds organic sweet potatoes

¼ cup coconut oil

½ teaspoon sea salt

1 tablespoon minced organic garlic

2 tablespoons Frontier brand organic adobo

2½ teaspoons Frontier brand muchi curry powder

Preheat the oven to 450°F. Slice the potatoes lengthwise into long strips, about ½-inch thick and about 5 inches long. Place the fries in a large bowl. (If you don't have your gloves on yet, now is a good time to put them on.)

Drizzle the coconut oil over the fries, and mix with your hands to ensure an even coating. Add the sea salt, garlic, and adobo and mix well, making sure all fries are coated. Add the curry powder and mix again.

Place a sheet of unbleached parchment paper on a large baking sheet. Place a stainless-steel cooling rack on top.

Place handfuls of fries on the rack and spread them out evenly, making sure they are not on top of one another. Place the baking sheet in the oven on the middle rack and bake for 25 minutes. Remove from the oven. Using tongs, flip the fries over and bake for another 4 to 6 minutes.

Remove the fries from the oven and allow to cool for 5 minutes before taking them off the rack.

DESSERTS

Overnight Vanilla Oats and Chia

This is my version of pudding, which makes an after-dinner treat. It has a wonderful texture and tastes similar to rice or tapioca pudding. It is a great dessert that the whole family will love!

1 cup coconut-almond milk

2 tablespoons organic chia seeds

⅓ cup gluten-free oats

2 teaspoons coconut nectar or ½ teaspoon lo-han sweetener

1 teaspoon vanilla extract, alcohol-free

½ teaspoon organic ground cinnamon

Slivered almonds

Organic blueberries

In an 8- to 10-ounce mason jar, combine the milk, chia seeds, oats, coconut nectar, vanilla, and cinnamon and stir well. Cover and refrigerate overnight. Top with almonds and blueberries before serving.

Coconut Yogurt Parfait

½ cup Anita's Creamline Coconut Yogurt

¼ cup mixed organic berries

2 tablespoons slivered toasted organic almonds

2 to 3 tablespoons Vanilla-Coconut Whipped Cream (page 321)

Place the yogurt in a small dish, then top with the berries, almonds, and coconut whipped cream. If you prefer it a bit sweeter, add a pinch of lo-han or stevia to the yogurt and mix to incorporate. Serve chilled.

Chia Pudding Deluxe with Mango

1½ cups vanilla-coconut blend milk

4 tablespoons organic chia seeds

1 tablespoon coconut nectar

½ teaspoon lo-han sweetener

⅛ teaspoon Himalayan pink sea salt

½ teaspoon organic ground cinnamon

1 vanilla bean pod, split and seeds scraped

¾ cup chopped organic mango

Fresh organic berries, for garnish

In a small bowl, combine the milk and chia seeds and stir. Set aside for 30 minutes. The mixture will thicken. After 30 minutes, place the chia mixture, coconut nectar, lo-han, salt, cinnamon, and vanilla in a Vitamix or other heavy-duty blender and blend on high for 1 minute. The pudding should be smooth but not completely puréed. Serve chilled in small bowls and garnish with fresh berries.

Vanilla-Coconut Whipped Cream

MAKES ABOUT 1 CUP

1 can (13.5 ounces) full-fat coconut milk (Natural Value or Native
  Forest brand; chilled in refrigerator for 24 hours)
1 teaspoon lo-han sweetener or a pinch or two of stevia
2 teaspoons vanilla extract, alcohol-free

About an hour or so before making the whipped cream, chill a stainless-steel bowl in the freezer. Next, flip the chilled can of coconut milk upside down and open it. Drain the liquid into a cup and save for shakes, smoothies, or stews, if you like. Transfer the solid coconut milk into the chilled bowl and beat with an electric mixer until peaks form and it doubles in volume. Add the sweetener and vanilla and continue to mix. It should resemble traditional whipped cream.

Cover and refrigerate immediately if you will not be consuming within 15 minutes.

Ultimate Immune Lollipop

. . . .

MAKES 4 SERVINGS

What kid doesn't love a lollipop? Well, you don't have to be a kid to enjoy these immune-boosting lollipops. The vitamin C and elderberry are great for supporting your immune system and warding off upper respiratory infections. And they taste good, too!

½ cup organic cherries (frozen is best; defrost for 2 hours)

⅔ cup cherry juice (from defrosted cherries)

1 teaspoon lo-han syrup

1 tablespoon filtered water

1 teaspoon organic lime juice

1 teaspoon full-fat Califia Farms organic coconut milk

1 scoop buffered vitamin C powder (Thorne)

4 teaspoons Gaia Herbs brand black elderberry syrup

1 teaspoon grated fresh organic ginger

Place all of the ingredients into a Vitamix or other heavy-duty blender and blend on high for 1 to 2 minutes. Pour into an ice-pop mold and freeze according to the manufacturer's directions.

BEVERAGES

Fatigue-Fighting Green Thyme Tea

MAKES 2 SERVINGS

If you are trying to kick your coffee habit, try starting your day by drinking this instead. Green tea is a potent antioxidant and can help protect against heart disease, cancer, and inflammation. Since it does contain a small amount of caffeine, I recommend drinking it before three p.m., so it doesn't interfere with your sleep.

4 cups filtered water

2 teaspoons organic dried thyme or 4 teaspoons fresh thyme

1 heaping teaspoon of good-quality loose green tea

In a teakettle or medium saucepan, bring the water to a boil. Place the thyme and green tea in a teapot with a strainer or tea infuser and pour the boiling water over it. Cover and allow to steep for 5 minutes. Strain and serve. Add a squeeze of lemon if you like.

Hydrating Watermelon, Pear, and Mint Drink

MAKES 2 SERVINGS

When I think of watermelon, I think of summer. This cool, refreshing drink is great for those hot summer days when you just want to relax and rehydrate yourself. I'll even add a splash of freshly squeezed lime juice to give it more flavor.

8 ounces organic watermelon juice

4 ounces chopped organic watermelon

6 sprigs organic mint leaves

8 ounces filtered water

½ organic pear, peeled and chopped

Place all of the ingredients in a Vitamix or other heavy-duty blender and blend until smooth.

Resources

Air Purifiers

Austin Air: *austinair.com*
Blueair: *blueair.com*
E. L. Foust: *foustco.com*
IQAir: *iqair.com*

Community

Darin Ingels, ND: *dariningelsnd.com*
Facebook: *facebook.com/DarinIngelsND* and *facebook.com/LymeExpertND*
Instagram: *instagram.com/dariningelsnd*
Twitter: *twitter.com/DrDarinIngels* and *twitter.com/lymeexpertND*
YouTube: *YouTube.com/DarinIngelsND*

Counseling and Support

Audrey Amir, LMSW: *audreyamir.com*
Lyme Disease Network: *lymenet.org/SupportGroups/UnitedStates/*
Lymedisease.org (USA): *lymedisease.org/get-involved/take-action/
    find-your-state-group/*
Lymedisease.org (Australia): *lymedisease.org.au/resources/*
Lyme Disease Support Network: *lymediseasesupportnetwork.org/users*
Tired of Lyme: *tiredoflyme.com/online-support-groups.html*

Homeopathy

Cindy Chrisman, CCH: *homeopathicprovider.com*
Julia Eastman, LAc, CCH: *juliaaeastman.com*
Lisette Narragon, CCH: *bayareahomeopathy.com*
National Center for Homeopathy: *homeopathycenter.org*

Immunotherapy Practitioners

American Academy of Allergy, Asthma, and Immunology: *aaaai.org*
American Academy of Environmental Medicine: *aaemonline.org*
Ty Vincent, MD: *globalimmunotherapy.com*
Wellness Integrative Naturopathic Center: *wellnessintegrative.com*

Integrative Medicine Practitioners (Lyme-Literate)

American Academy of Environmental Medicine: *aaemonline.org*
American Association of Integrative Medicine: *aaimedicine.com*
American Association of Naturopathic Physicians: *naturopathic.org*
Institute for Functional Medicine: *functionalmedicine.org*
International Lyme and Associated Diseases Society: *ilads.org*

Mold Inspection and Testing

Please search for a local mold inspector who can offer spore trapping, ERMI testing, and direct sampling for visible mold.

Natural Cleaning Products

Bon Ami: *bonami.com/index.php/products/powder_cleanser/*
Debra Lynn Dadd: *debralynndadd.com/debras-list/selected-toxic-free -products/*
Earth Friendly Products: *ecos.com*
Ecover: *us.ecover.com*
Environmental Working Group: *ewg.org/guides/cleaners/content/top _products*
Greening the Cleaning: *greeningthecleaning.com*
Planet: *planetinc.com*
Safer Chemicals, Healthy Families: *saferchemicals.org*

Seventh Generation: *seventhgeneration.com*
Whole Foods: *wholefoodsmarket.com*

Natural Personal-Care Products

Campaign for Safe Cosmetics: *safecosmetics.org*
Debra Lynn Dadd: *debralynndadd.com/debras-list/selected-toxic-free-products/*
Dr. Bronner's: *drbronner.com*
Environmental Working Group: *ewg.org*
Organic Consumers Association: *organicconsumers.org/old_articles
   /bodycare/links.php*
Tom's of Maine: *tomsofmaine.com/home*

Nutritional Support

Annalyce Loretto: *thethoughtfulkitchen.com*
Clara Barnett, ND, Lac: *drclara.com*
Shanel Sinclair: *augustastreetkitchen.com*

Laboratory Testing

Commonwealth Laboratories: *hydrogenbreathtesting.com*
Cyrex Laboratories: *cyrexlabs.com*
Doctor's Data: *doctorsdata.com*
Genova Diagnostics: *gdx.net*
Great Plains Laboratory: *greatplainslaboratory.com*
Immunosciences Lab: *immunoscienceslab.com*
Laboratory Corporation of America (LabCorp): *labcorp.com/wps/portal*
Quest Diagnostics: *questdiagnostics.com/home.html*
SpectraCell Laboratories: *spectracell.com*
RealTime Laboratories: *realtimelab.com*

Lyme Laboratory Testing

Armin Labs: *arminlabs.com/en*
Global Lyme Diagnostics: *glymedx.com*
IGeneX: *igenex.com*
Medical Diagnostic Laboratories: *mdlab.com*

Pulsed Electromagnetic Frequency (PEMF) Devices

Bemer: *united-states.bemergroup.com/en-US*
Lenyosys: *lenyosys.com*

Supplements

Please visit our online store at *dariningelsnd.com*.

Water Purifiers

Aquasana: *aquasana.com*
E. L. Foust: *foustco.com*
Rainshow'r: *rainshowermfg.com*

Appendix A. Lyme and Co-Infections

This book is designed to help you navigate Lyme disease, but when you get a tick bite, you may also get other infections in addition to Lyme. Many ticks that carry Lyme disease also carry a host of other infections that can be transmitted through the same bite. To make things more confusing, many of the symptoms of Lyme disease can be caused by these other infections, so it is difficult to distinguish what is related to Lyme disease from what is coming from some other infection. So when you get tested for Lyme disease (see Chapter 2), it is a good idea to test for all of the co-infections at the same time, so you and your doctor can be clear on what you are treating.

Every year, it seems, I read more and more about the discovery of new bacteria and viruses that can be transmitted through a tick bite. We used to think it was only a handful of bugs, but we now know that potentially hundreds of different microbes can infect humans and make you sick. Some of the more common co-infections include the following:

BARTONELLA

This bacterium is mostly known as a cause of "cat scratch fever." As the name suggests, you can get this from being scratched by a cat, but it is transmitted through ticks as well. The most common organism is *Bartonella henselae*, but at least eight species found in humans cause disease. One of the telltale symptoms of *Bartonella* is the presence of a rash that looks like stretch marks, found mostly on the back, abdomen, and arms. These red streaks often start to appear after people begin to feel sick and are unrelated to weight loss. Other symptoms of *Bartonella* include fatigue, swollen lymph nodes, numbness or tingling, headaches, joint or muscle pain, and insomnia.

BABESIA

This parasite gets inside your red blood cells and is a close cousin of malaria. *Babesia microti* and *Babesia duncani* are the two species we find most in infected people. Since it is a blood parasite, it can be transmitted through a blood transfusion as well as a tick bite. Babesia can cause many symptoms similar to Lyme disease, but some of the symptoms more specific to *Babesia* are a cyclical high fever (also seen in malaria), profuse sweating, chest pain, shortness of breath ("air hunger"), and hip pain.

In more severe cases, *Babesia* can lead to a condition called hemolytic anemia, where the parasites cause your red blood cells to break down and can make your skin and eyes turn yellow (called jaundice). As your red blood cells break down, they are less able to carry oxygen, so you can feel short of breath, even when you are not exerting yourself. *Babesia* can also cause severe low blood pressure and liver failure if left untreated. Elderly people and those with a compromised immune system are most at risk of having complications—which can even be fatal—with *Babesia*.[1]

ANAPLASMA

The bacterium *Anaplasma phagocytophilum* causes symptoms similar to Lyme disease and has no characteristic symptoms that distinguish it from other tick-borne infections. However, this organism can infect white blood cells, so you may find that your white count is lower than expected when you run a blood test.

EHRLICHIA

The bacterium *Ehrlichia chaffeensis* is responsible for most *Ehrlichia* infections in the United States. It is very similar to *Anaplasma* and causes comparable symptoms. Like *Anaplasma*, it can also cause your white blood cell count to drop.

RICKETTSIA

Rickettsia is associated with Rocky Mountain spotted fever. More than 90 percent of people who get infected with *Rickettsia rickettsii* develop a whole-body spotted rash that is different from the single bull's-eye rash caused by Lyme disease. However, other symptoms are similar to those of Lyme disease and, aside from the rash, can make it difficult to differentiate between the two.

Q FEVER

Found throughout the United States, this Lyme-like illness caused by *Coxiella burnetii* is transmitted through different ticks from those that transmit Lyme disease. Common symptoms include fever, chills, muscle aches, fatigue, and intestinal problems, but joint pain is rare with Q fever.

MYCOPLASMA

This is the primary agent responsible for "walking pneumonia," in which you feel tired and have a dry, hacking cough that seems to go on for weeks or longer. It is caused by *Mycoplasma pneumoniae* and is usually spread by someone coughing or sneezing on you but can also be transmitted by a tick bite. Some people who get mycoplasma through a tick bite never get a respiratory illness but can experience joint pain, fatigue, headaches, and inflammation in the eyes.

STARI

STARI (southern tick-associated rash illness) looks a lot like Lyme disease and causes a similar-looking but smaller bull's-eye rash. Deer ticks do not transmit it, but Lone Star ticks found throughout the eastern, southeastern, and south-central United States do. We do not know what causes STARI, but some experts believe it is another species of *Borrelia* that has yet to be identified.

Many other microbes can be transmitted by a tick bite, so if you have Lyme-like symptoms and all of your tests keep coming up negative, it is a good idea to talk with your doctor to test for these other bugs that may be making you sick. Some of the other illnesses that look like Lyme disease include Powassan virus, Colorado tick fever, tularemia, and relapsing tick fever.

Appendix B. Current CDC Guidelines for the Treatment of Lyme Disease

My hope for you in reading this book is that you don't ever have to use any of these protocols. But I think it's good to know what is typically recommended, so you can have a meaningful discussion with your doctor about the best course of action in treating your Lyme. You'll notice that these recommendations have not been updated in more than a decade—but that's not altogether surprising, given that many conventional doctors cannot readily recognize Lyme as a potential cause of your symptoms, nor do they treat it as urgently as is warranted.

The current guidelines in the United States established by the Infectious Diseases Society of America (IDSA) in 2006 are as follows:[1]

Acute Tick Bite (Within 72 Hours of Bite)
- Adults or children over age eight: a single dose of 200 milligrams of doxycycline (however, there is no evidence this is effective)
- Children under age eight: no recommendations

Early-Onset Lyme Disease
- Adults: doxycycline (100 milligrams twice per day), amoxicillin (500 milligrams three times per day), or cefuroxime axetil (500 milligrams twice per day) for 14 to 21 days
- Children over age eight: doxycycline (4 mg/kg per day in two divided doses) up to 100 milligrams per dose
- Children under age eight: amoxicillin (50 mg/kg per day in three divided doses) up to 500 milligrams per dose, or cefuroxime axetil (30 mg/kg per day in two divided doses) up to 500 milligrams per dose

Lyme Meningitis or Early Neurological Disease
- Adults: ceftriaxone (2 grams once per day intravenously for 14 to 28 days) or cefotaxime (2 grams intravenously every eight hours) or penicillin G (18 to 24 million U per day every four hours)
- Children: ceftriaxone (50 to 75 mg/kg per day) in a single daily intravenous dose (maximum 2 grams) is the treatment of choice. Otherwise, cefotaxime (150 to 200 mg/kg per day) divided into three or four intravenous doses per day (maximum 6 grams) or penicillin G (200,000 to 400,000 units/kg per day up to 18 to 24 million U per day) given intravenously every four hours

Late Neurological Lyme Disease
- Adults and children: intravenous ceftriaxone for 2 to 4 weeks is preferable. Cefotaxime or penicillin G administered intravenously may also be used. Doses are the same as in early neurological disease.

Post-Lyme-Disease Syndrome
- Adults and children—no treatment recommendations

Appendix C. Autoimmune Diseases

Although more than a hundred conditions are associated with autoimmune disease, here are some of the more common ones, many of which have no known triggers. Having one of the following diseases could suggest that Lyme disease or another infectious disease is the root problem:

- Alopecia (hair loss)
- Dermatomyositis
- Diabetes (type 1)
- Glomerulonephritis
- Graves' disease (hyperthyroid)
- Guillain-Barré syndrome
- Hashimoto's disease (hypothyroid)
- Hemolytic anemia
- Hepatitis (autoimmune type)
- Idiopathic thrombocytopenic purpura
- Juvenile arthritis
- Myasthenia gravis
- Myocarditis (autoimmune type)
- Multiple sclerosis
- Pemphigus/pemphigoid
- Pernicious anemia
- Polyarteritis nodosa
- Polymyositis
- Primary biliary cirrhosis

- Psoriasis
- Rheumatoid arthritis
- Scleroderma
- Sjögren's syndrome
- Systemic lupus erythematosus
- Uveitis (autoimmune type)
- Vitiligo

If you have any of these conditions, you may want to talk with your doctor about getting tested for Lyme disease and co-infections, as they may be an underlying cause to your illness.

Acknowledgments

Writing this book could not have been accomplished without the help of many, many people along the way. I have been blessed to have so many good people in my life who helped make this book possible.

This book is for all of my brothers and sisters in the fight with me against Lyme disease. I have walked in your shoes, and I hope that you can find the path to recovery as I have.

I have to say a special "Thank you" to Amy Myers, MD, who really helped get the ball rolling for this book. I was fortunate enough to meet Amy at a conference where we were both speaking, and she was kind enough to help guide me on making this book happen. Thank you for your friendship and willingness to help me navigate the world of publishing.

Thanks to my agent, Stephanie Tade, who was able to see the vision of this book. You made this process easier than imaginable and put me in touch with the right people to help tell my story and share my experience to help others with Lyme disease.

Thanks to all of the staff at Avery who believed in me and agreed to publish my work. I am especially grateful to Caroline Sutton and Brianna Flaherty for their constructive feedback and help in bringing the book to life. Thanks, too, to Megan Newman, Lindsay Gordon, Farin Schlussel, Allyssa Kasoff, Emily Fisher, and Hannah Steigmeyer.

I am especially grateful to Alison Rose Levy, with whom I share this book as my collaborator, for you were able to express my thoughts in ways that I could never have imagined.

Thank you, Shanel Sinclair, for helping develop our recipes and coming up with creative ways to make changing one's diet easy and delicious. Your dedication to healthy, allergy-free foods is inspiring, and it shows in everything you make.

While writing this book, I was working full time and running multiple practices. I couldn't have managed the time I needed to write this book without the tireless effort of my team at Ingels Family Health and Wellness Integrative Naturopathic Center to keep everything running smoothly and taking such good care of our patients. Special thanks to Gloria Terrell, who had been hounding me to write a book for years; Dr. Mark Sanders; Dr. Nina Manipon; Dr. Jill Kenney; Cindy Wechsler, APRN; Maggie White; Ellen Demotses; Amy Delardi; Yoana Brecker; Tania Lenna; Anabel Aguilar; and Wendy Frost.

And I thank all of my patients who have entrusted their care to me over the years. You ultimately are my teachers and help me become a better doctor. I learn from you and the experiences you share with me. You are the reason I come to work every day as we work together toward better health.

My medical career started at Lutheran General Hospital in Park Ridge, Illinois, working as a clinical microbiologist/immunologist, and I was fortunate to have some amazing mentors who really taught me about microbes and disease, especially Lynn Dusing, Sharon Petree, Dr. Mike Costello, Dr. Nik Bharani, Dr. Takashi Okuno, and Dr. Imad Almanaseer. Thank you for teaching me how to be a good clinical pathologist.

I have been fortunate in my career to work with kind, compassionate, brilliant doctors who have mentored me and helped me grow as a doctor: my good friends and colleagues Dr. Kelly McCann, Dr. Jerry Kartzinel, Dr. Anju Usman, Dr. Carrie Ganek, Dr. Melissa Macfarlane, Dr. Clara Barnett, Dr. Peter Bongiorno, Dr. Pina LoGiudice, Dr. Alan Gaby, Dr. Jonathan Goodman, Dr. Deborah Metzger, Dr. Larry Palevsky, Dr. Kasra Pournadeali, and Dr. Ty Vincent. Special thanks to Mary Coyle for years of friendship and collaboration with complex cases.

I also thank my friends and family, who have been a great source of support and laughter. My parents, Joe and Kamy, are always there for me and taught me to be the man I am today. I am also grateful to my sister, Jen, and her husband, Jon; my brother, Jon; and my aunt Kathy. I couldn't have made it through the tough times without the friendship of Chris and Jackie Raimann, who always knew how to make me laugh and keep life in perspective. Thank you to my other "Village" friends, Pete and Amy Delardi, Chris and Sue Waters, and Carlo and Katie Romeo, for always being willing to lend a helping hand when needed.

Most important, I want to thank my dear, sweet Dr. Jessica Tran. You are my partner in business and life. Your love, support, and being a sounding board for my ideas made this book possible. Thank you for your patience with all the craziness in our world. I love you.

Notes

CHAPTER 1: WHY ANTIBIOTICS AREN'T ENOUGH

1. **identified in more than eighty countries around the world:** lymediseaseassocia tion.org/about-lyme/cases-stats-maps-a-graphs/940-lyme-in-more-than-80 -countries-worldwide.

2. **Warmer weather increases the mice population:** npr.org/sections/goatsandsoda /2017/03/06/518219485/forbidding-forecast-for-lyme-disease-in-the-northeast.

3. **Rising global temperatures will exacerbate the trend toward more insect-borne diseases:** World Health Organization. (2016). *All about climate change and vector borne diseases.* wpro.who.int/mvp/climate_change/en/; McIver L, Kim R, Wood ward A, et al. (2016). Health impacts of climate change in Pacific Island countries: a regional assessment of vulnerabilities and adaptation priorities. *Environ Health Perspect* 124 (11): 1707–1714. doi.org/10.1289/ehp.1509756.

4. **evidence suggests it has been around for thousands of years:** Summerton N. (1995). Lyme disease in the eighteenth century. *BMJ* 311 (7018): 1478. doi:10.1136 /bmj.311.7018.1478.

5. **"Ötzi the Iceman," a 5,300-year-old mummy found in the Austrian Alps:** Hall SS. (November 2011). Iceman autopsy. *Nat Geog Mag.* ngm.nationalgeographic .com/2011/11/iceman-autopsy/hall-text.

6. **suggesting some type of bacteria had caused the arthritis:** Steere AC, Malawista SE, Bartenhagen NH, et al. (1984). The clinical spectrum and treatment of Lyme disease. *Yale J Biol Med* 57 (4): 453–464.

7. **the fastest-growing insect-borne infectious disease in the United States, Europe, and Asia:** Qiu W-G, Bruno JF, McCaig WD, et al. (2008). Wide distribution of a high-virulence *Borrelia burgdorferi* clone in Europe and North America. *Emerg*

Infect Dis 14 (7): 1097–1104. doi.org/10.3201/eid1407.070880; Geographic distribution and expansion of human Lyme disease, United States. (2015). *Emerg Infect Dis* 21 (8): 1455–1457. doi.org/10.3201/eid2108.141878; Marques AR. (2010). Lyme disease: a review. *Curr Allergy Asthma Rep* 10 (1): 13–20. doi:10.1007/s11882-009-0077-3.

8. **many more cases go unreported or are undiagnosed:** Berger S. (2014). *Lyme disease: Global Status 2014 Edition* (Los Angeles: Gideon Informatics), 7.

9. **unless antibiotics are administered within seventy-two hours of a deer tick bite, they have a poor track record:** nejm.org/doi/full/10.1056/NEJM200107123450201#t=article.

10. **up to two thirds of people with Lyme disease will fail conventional antibiotic therapy:** Stricker RB, Johnson L. (2016). Lyme disease: the promise of Big Data, companion diagnostics and precision medicine. *Infect Drug Resist* 9: 215–219. doi.org/10.2147/IDR.S114770.

11. **can change its shape to hide from your immune system:** Meriläinen L, Herranen A, Schwarzbach A, Gilbert L. (2015). Morphological and biochemical features of *Borrelia burgdorferi* pleomorphic forms. *Microbiol* 161 (Pt 3), 516–527. doi.org/10.1099/mic.0.000027.

12. **Lyme spirochetes can hide in your lymph nodes:** www.sciencedaily.com/releases/2011/06/110616193911.htm; google.com/webhp?sourceid=chrome-instant&rlz=1C1CHWA_enUS609US609&ion=1&espv=2&ie=UTF-8#q=:+Lyme+spirochetes+can+hide+in+your+lymph+nodes.

13. *Borrelia* **can literally coil itself into a ball:** ncbi.nlm.nih.gov/pmc/articles/PMC2774030/.

14. **treating Lyme disease of the brain:** Miklossy J, Kasas S, Zurn AD, McCall S, Yu S, McGeer PL. (2008). Persisting atypical and cystic forms of *Borrelia burgdorferi* and local inflammation in Lyme neuroborreliosis. *J Neuroinflammation* 5: 40. doi.org/10.1186/1742-2094-5-40.

15. *Borrelia burgdorferi,* **with fifteen subspecies, causes most of the cases of Lyme disease in the United States:** Baum E, Hue F, Barbour AG. (2012). Experimental infections of the reservoir *Peromyscus leucopus* with diverse strains of *Borrelia burgdorferi*, a Lyme disease agent. *MBio* 3 (6): e00434–12.

16. **common species responsible for Lyme disease in the United States and Europe:** Tilly K, Rosa PA, Stewart PE. (2008). Biology of infection with *Borrelia burgdorferi*. *Infect Dis Clin North Am* 22 (2): 217–234. doi.org/10.1016/j.idc.2007.12.013.

17. **genetic differences between the Lyme bacteria found in the United States and those found in Europe:** Cerar T, Strle F, Stupica D, et al. (2016). Differences in genotype, clinical features, and inflammatory potential of *Borrelia burgdorferi* sensu stricto strains from Europe and the United States. *Emerg Infect Dis* 22 (5): 818–827. doi.org/10.3201/eid2205.151806; Baum E, Hue F, Barbour AG. (2012). Experimental infections of the reservoir *Peromyscus leucopus* with diverse strains of *Borrelia burgdorferi*, a Lyme disease agent. *MBio* 3 (6): e00434–12.

18. **ticks must be attached to your skin for thirty-six to forty-eight hours:** Centers for Disease Control. (2016). Lyme disease: transmission. cdc.gov/lyme/transmission/.

19. **some ticks can transmit Lyme disease within sixteen hours:** Shih CM, Spielman A. (1993). Accelerated transmission of Lyme disease spirochetes by partially fed vector ticks. *J Clin Microbiol* 31 (11): 2878–2881.

20. **mothers with Lyme disease have a higher rate of complications at birth:** Williams CL, Strobino B, Weinstein A, Spierling P, Medici F. (1995). Maternal Lyme disease and congenital malformations: a cord blood serosurvey in endemic and control areas. *Paediatr Perinat Epidemiol* 9 (3): 320–330; Larsson C, Andersson M, Guo BP, et al. (2006). Complications of pregnancy and transplacental transmission of relapsing-fever borreliosis. *J Infect Dis* 194 (10): 1367–1374.

21. **destruction of friendly bacteria creates a disrupted gut ecology, making your immune system less efficient in getting rid of infections:** Mariño E. (2016). The gut microbiota and immune-regulation: the fate of health and disease. *Clin Transl Immunol* 5 (11): e107. doi.org/10.1038/cti.2016.61; Levy M, Blacher E, Elinav E. (2016). Microbiome, metabolites and host immunity. *Curr Opin Microbiol* 35: 8–15. doi:10.1016/j.mib.2016.10.003; Filyk HA, Osborne LC. (2016). The multibiome: the intestinal ecosystem's influence on immune homeostasis, health, and disease. *EBioMedicine* 13: 46–54. doi:10.1016/j.ebiom.2016.10.007.

22. **and go on to develop post-treatment Lyme disease syndrome:** Centers for Disease Control and Prevention. (2016). Post-treatment Lyme Disease Syndrome. cdc.gov/lyme/postLDS/index.html

23. **persister bacteria have developed clever ways of altering hundreds of their genes:** Feng J, Shi W, Zhang S, Zhang Y. (2015). Persister mechanisms in *Borrelia burgdorferi*: implications for improved intervention. *Emerg Microbes Infect* 4 (8): e51. doi.org/10.1038/emi.2015.51.

24. **the persister bacteria seem to survive because they grow at a slower rate:** Caskey JR, Embers ME. (2015). Persister development by *Borrelia burgdorferi* populations in vitro. *Antimicrob Agents Chemother* 59 (10): 6288–6295. doi.org/10.1128/AAC .00883–15.

25. **certain antibiotics are better than others at eliminating persister bacteria:** Feng J, Wang T, Shi W, et al. (2014). Identification of novel activity against *Borrelia burgdorferi* persisters using an FDA approved drug library. *Emerg Microbes Infect* 3 (7): e49. doi.org/10.1038/emi.2014.53.

26. **the Lyme spirochete replicates every one to sixteen days:** Jutras BL, Chenail AM, Stevenson B. (2013). Changes in bacterial growth rate govern expression of the *Borrelia burgdorferi* OspC and Erp infection-associated surface proteins. *J Bacteriol* 195 (4): 757–764. doi.org/10.1128/JB.01956–12.

27. **no difference between the treatment groups and the placebo group:** Berende A, ter Hofstede HJ, Vos FJ, et al. (2016). Randomized trial of longer-term therapy for symptoms attributed to Lyme disease. *N Engl J Med* 374 (13): 1209–1220. doi:10.1056/NEJMoa1505425.

28. **two drugs commonly used to treat Lyme, were unable to kill persistent *Borrelia burgdorferi*:** Feng J, Weitner M, Shi W, Zhang S, Zhang Y. (2016). Eradication of biofilm-like microcolony structures of *Borrelia burgdorferi* by daunomycin and daptomycin but not mitomycin C in combination with doxycycline and cefuroxime. Front Microbiol 7: 62. doi.org/10.3389/fmicb.2016.00062.

29. **people with post-treatment Lyme disease of the brain had mild cognitive improvement:** Fallon BA, Keilp JG, Corbera KM, et al. (2008). A randomized, placebo-controlled trial of repeated IV antibiotic therapy for Lyme encephalopathy. *Neurology* 70 (13): 992–1003.

30. **the International Lyme and Associated Diseases Society (ILADS) developed guidelines for treating Lyme disease that are radically different:** Cameron DJ, Johnson LB, Maloney EL. (2014). Evidence assessments and guideline recommendations in Lyme disease: the clinical management of known tick bites, erythema migrans rashes and persistent disease. *Expert Rev Anti Infect Ther* 12 (9): 1103–1135. doi.org/10.1586/14787210.2014.940900.

31. **Autoimmune diseases have steadily been on the rise:** Lerner A, Jeremias P, Matthias T. (2015). The world incidence and prevalence of autoimmune diseases is increasing. *Int J Celiac Dis* 3 (4): 1511–1155.

32. **more than 120 different diseases are either known or suspected to be related to autoimmunity:** aarda.org/autoimmune-information/autoimmune-statistics/.

33. **increase in autoimmune disease almost parallels the rise in asthma and allergies:** Okada H, Kuhn C, Feillet H, Bach J-F. (2010). The "hygiene hypothesis" for autoimmune and allergic diseases: an update. *Clin Exp Immunol* 160 (1): 1–9. doi.org/10.1111/j.1365-2249.2010.04139.x.

34. **bacteria and viruses may sometimes cause the immune system to start working against itself:** ncbi.nlm.nih.gov/pmc/articles/PMC2665673/.

35. **scientists suggest that T cells accidentally make two receptors:** Cusick MF, Libbey JE, Fujinami RS. (2012). Molecular mimicry as a mechanism of autoimmune disease. *Clin Rev Allergy Immunol* 42 (1): 102–111. doi.org/10.1007/s12016-011-8293-8.

36. **outer-surface protein A (OspA), is structurally similar to a protein in our body:** Steere AC, Gross D, Meyer AL, Huber BT. (2001). Autoimmune mechanisms in antibiotic treatment-resistant lyme arthritis. *J Autoimmun* 16 (3): 263–268.

37. **Multiple other proteins also cross-react with the Lyme organism:** Pianta A, Drouin EE, Crowley JT, et al. (2015). Annexin A2 is a target of autoimmune T and B cell responses associated with synovial fibroblast proliferation in patients with antibiotic-refractory Lyme arthritis. *Clin Immunol (Orlando, Fla.)* 160 (2): 336–341. doi.org/10.1016/j.clim.2015.07.005.

38. **antibodies directed against the tail (called the *flagellum*) of the Lyme disease bacterium cross-react with a protein in the nerves:** Sigal LH, Williams S. (1997). A monoclonal antibody to *Borrelia burgdorferi* flagellin modifies neuroblastoma

cell neuritogenesis in vitro: a possible role for autoimmunity in the neuropathy of Lyme disease. *Infect Immun* 65 (5): 1722–1728.

39. **Lyme-reactive antibodies form against proteins in the brain:** Kaiser R. (1995). Intrathecal immune response in patients with neuroborreliosis: specificity of antibodies for neuronal proteins. *J Neurol* 242 (5): 319–325.

CHAPTER 2: HOW DO YOU KNOW IF YOU HAVE LYME?

1. **70 to 80 percent of people with Lyme disease get the bull's-eye rash:** cdc.gov /lyme/signs_symptoms/.

2. **the rash may be seen in only up to 50 percent of people who get Lyme disease:** ilads.org/lyme/about-lyme.php; Donta ST. (2002). Late and chronic Lyme disease. *Med Clin North Am* 86 (2):341–349, vii.

3. **Joint swelling, another sign of Lyme disease, is not a reliable gauge either:** Bacon RM, Kugeler KJ, Mead PS; Centers for Disease Control and Prevention (CDC). (2008). Surveillance for Lyme disease—United States, 1992–2006. *MMWR Surveill Summ* 57 (10): 1–9.

4. *Borrelia miyomotoi:* Nelder MP, Russell CB, Sheehan NJ, et al. (2016). Human pathogens associated with the blacklegged tick *Ixodes scapularis*: a systematic review. *Parasit Vectors* 9: 265. doi.org/10.1186/s13071-016-1529-y.

5. *Borrelia garinii:* https://wwwnc.cdc.gov/eid/article/22/5/pdfs/15-1806.pdf.

6. *Borrelia afzelii:* Ibid.

7. *Borrelia mayonii:* www.cdc.gov/ticks/mayonii.html.

8. *Borrelia lonestari:* James AM, Liveris D, Wormser GP, Schwartz I, Montecalvo MA, Johnson BJB. (2001). *Borrelia lonestari* infection after a bite by an *Amblyomma americanum* tick. *J Infect Dis* 83 (12): 1810–1814. doi:10.1086/320721.

9. **countless people who were told by doctors that they didn't have Lyme disease because they never developed it:** Johnson L, Wilson S, Mankoff J, Stricker RB. (2014) Severity of chronic Lyme disease compared to other chronic conditions: a quality of life survey. *PeerJ* 2: e322. doi.org/10.7717/peerj.322.

10. **Other current tests can miss up to 60 percent of Lyme cases:** Stricker RB, Johnson L. (2016). Lyme disease: the promise of Big Data, companion diagnostics and precision medicine. *Infect Drug Resist* 9: 215–219. doi.org/10.2147/IDR .S114770.

11. **currently available tests for the Lyme spirochete as no more effective than tossing a coin:** Stricker RB, Johnson L. (2007). Let's tackle the testing. *BMJ* 335 (7628): 1008. doi.org/10.1136/bmj.39394.676227.BE.

12. **in fifty-five people with known Lyme disease, less than 46 percent of them had either IgG or IgM antibodies:** Engstrom SM, Shoop E, Johnson RC. (1995). Immunoblot interpretation criteria for serodiagnosis of early Lyme disease. *J Clin Microbiol* 33: 419–427.

13. **The Lyme screen test does not meet these criteria:** Bakken LL, Callister SM, Wand PJ, Schell RF. (1997). Interlaboratory comparison of test results for detection of Lyme disease by 516 participants in the Wisconsin State Laboratory of Hygiene/College of American Pathologists Proficiency Testing Program. *J Clin Microbiol* 35: 537–543.

14. **the Lyme screen test may only pick up about 56 percent of people who have Lyme disease:** Stricker RB, Johnson L. (2007). Let's tackle the testing. *BMJ* 335 (7628): 1008. doi.org/10.1136/bmj.39394.676227.BE.

15. **Western blot is more accurate in diagnosing Lyme disease because it looks for specific antibodies:** Ma B, Christen B, Leung D, Vigo-Pelfrey C. (1992). Serodiagnosis of Lyme borreliosis by Western immunoblot: reactivity of various significant antibodies against *Borrelia burgdorferi*. *J Clin Microbiol* 30 (2): 370–376.

16. **the criteria used to call a Western blot test "positive" are thirty years old:** Association of State and Territorial Public Health Laboratory Directors (ASTPHLD). (1994). Proceedings of the Second National Conference on the Serological Diagnosis of Lyme Disease, October 27–29, Dearborn, MI.

17. **less than 50 percent of people with active Lyme disease have a positive PCR test:** Waddell LA, Greig J, Mascarenhas M, Harding S, Lindsay R, Ogden N. (2016). The accuracy of diagnostic tests for Lyme disease in humans, a systematic review and meta-analysis of North American research. *PLoS ONE* 11 (12): e0168613. doi.org/10.1371/journal.pone.0168613.

18. **Increased levels of IgG may actually interfere with the PCR test:** Al-Soud WA, Rådström P. (2001). Purification and characterization of PCR-inhibitory components in blood cells. *J Clin Microbiol* 39 (2): 485–493. doi.org/10.1128/JCM.39.2.485-493.2001.

19. **That percentage is even lower for those with chronic Lyme:** Sapi E, Pabbati N, Datar A, Davies EM, Rattelle A, Kuo BA. (2013). Improved culture conditions for the growth and detection of *Borrelia* from human serum. *Int J Med Sci* 10 (4), 362–376. doi.org/10.7150/ijms.5698.

CHAPTER 3: THE GUT PROTOCOL THAT RESTORES YOUR IMMUNE SYSTEM

1. **Eating highly processed foods, taking antibiotics or other medications, stress, or genetic conditions like celiac disease:** Otani K, Tanigawa T, Watanabe T, et al. (2017). Microbiota plays a key role in non-steroidal anti-inflammatory drug-induced small intestinal damage. *Digestion* 95: 22–28. doi:10.1159/000452356.

2. **The trillions of microbes that live in your gut are there for three reasons:** Wang Y, Kasper LH. (2014). The role of microbiome in central nervous system disorders. *Brain Behav Immun* 38: 1–12. doi.org/10.1016/j.bbi.2013.12.015.

3. **It's not at all uncommon for this digestive distress to turn into a more serious condition:** Jarjour WN, Jeffries BD, Davis JS, Welch WJ, Mimura T, Winfield JB.

(1991). Autoantibodies to human stress proteins. A survey of various rheumatic and other inflammatory diseases. *Arthritis Rheum* 34: 1133–1138. doi:10.1002 /art.1780340909.

4. **more than 25 percent of people with acute Lyme disease had other digestive issues:** Zaidi SA, Singer C. (2002). Gastrointestinal and hepatic manifestations of tickborne diseases in the United States. *Clin Infect Dis* 34 (9): 12061–12062.

5. **Leaky gut has been associated with:** Slyepchenko A, Maes M, Machado-Vieira R, et al. (2016). Intestinal dysbiosis, gut hyperpermeability and bacterial translocation: missing links between depression, obesity and type 2 diabetes. *Curr Pharm Des* 22 (40): 6087–6106; Forsyth CB, Shannon KM, Kordower JH, et al. (2011). Increased intestinal permeability correlates with sigmoid mucosa alpha-synuclein staining and endotoxin exposure markers in early Parkinson's disease. *PLoS ONE* 6 (12): e28032. doi.org/10.1371/journal.pone.0028032; Du L, Kim JJ, Shen J, Dai N. (2016). Crosstalk between inflammation and ROCK/MLCK signaling pathways in gastrointestinal disorders with intestinal hyperpermeability. *Gastroenterol Res Pract* 2016: 7374197. doi.org/10.1155/2016/7374197; Ito Y, Sasaki M, Funaki Y, et al. (2013). Nonsteroidal anti-inflammatory drug-induced visible and invisible small intestinal injury. *J Clin Biochem Nutr* 53 (1): 55–59. doi.org/10.3164/jcbn.121116.

6. **Diet is a major contributor to leaky gut. It has also been linked to drinking too much alcohol:** Engen PA, Green SJ, Voigt RM, Forsyth CB, Keshavarzian A. (2015). The gastrointestinal microbiome: alcohol effects on the composition of intestinal microbiota. *Alcohol Res* 37 (2): 223–236.

7. **eating a diet high in unhealthy fats, such as lard or cottonseed oil:** Murakami Y, Tanabe S, Suzuki T. (2016). High-fat diet-induced intestinal hyperpermeability is associated with increased bile acids in the large intestine of mice. *J Food Sci* 81 (1): H216–H222. doi:10.1111/17503–841.13166.

8. **Eating a low-fiber diet also seems to make leaky gut worse:** Desai MS, Seekatz AM, Koropatkin NM, et al. (2016). A dietary fiber-deprived gut microbiota degrades the colonic mucus barrier and enhances pathogen susceptibility. *Cell* 167 (5): 1339–1353.e21. doi:10.1016/j.ce.211016.10.043.

9. **Having an acidic gut doesn't help either:** Unno N, Hodin RA, Fink MP. (1999). Acidic conditions exacerbate interferon-gamma-induced intestinal epithelial hyperpermeability: role of peroxynitrous acid. *Crit Care Med* 27 (8): 1429–1436.

10. **The single best thing to help repair your gut, whether the damage was caused by dietary factors or using NSAIDS, is a good-quality probiotic:** Otani K, Tanigawa T, Watanabe T, et al. (2017). Microbiota plays a key role in non-steroidal anti-inflammatory drug-induced small intestinal damage. *Digestion* 95: 222–228 .doi:10.1159/000452356.

11. **studies show the beneficial effects of taking probiotics to rebuild a damaged gut wall:** Bron PA, Kleerebezem M, Brummer RJ, et al. (2017). Can probiotics modulate human disease by impacting intestinal barrier function? *Br J Nutr* 19: 11–15 .doi:10.1017/S0007114516004037.

12. **has been shown to help modulate inflammation and repair a leaky gut:** Khailova L, Baird CH, Rush AA, Barnes C, Wischmeyer PE. Lactobacillus rhamnosus GG treatment improves intestinal permeability and modulates inflammatory response and homeostasis of spleen and colon in experimental model of *Pseudomonas aeruginosa* pneumonia. *Clin Nutr* pii: S0261–5614(16)31265–1. doi:10.1016/j.clnu.2016.09.025.

13. **has been shown to help reduce inflammation that leads to leaky gut:** Krishnan M, Penrose HM, Shah NN, Marchelletta RR, McCole DF. (2016). VSL#3 probiotic stimulates T-cell protein tyrosine phosphatase-mediated recovery of IFN-γ-induced intestinal epithelial barrier defects. *Inflamm Bowel Dis* 22 (12): 2811–2823.

14. **These strains have all been shown to help protect the gut from infection and reduce inflammation:** Wu Y, Zhu C, Chen Z, et al. (2016). Protective effects of *Lactobacillus plantarum* on epithelial barrier disruption caused by enterotoxigenic *Escherichia coli* in intestinal porcine epithelial cells. *Vet Immunol Immunopathol* 172: 55–63. doi:10.1016/j.vetimm.2016.03.005; Srutkova D, Schwarzer M, Hudcovic T, et al. (2015). *Bifidobacterium longum* CCM 7952 promotes epithelial barrier function and prevents acute DSS-induced colitis in strictly strain-specific manner. *PLoS ONE* 10 (7): e0134050. doi.org/10.1371/journal.pone.0134050; Hummel S, Veltman K, Cichon C, Sonnenborn U, Schmidt MA. (2012). Differential targeting of the E-cadherin/β-catenin complex by gram-positive probiotic lactobacilli improves epithelial barrier function. *Applied Environ Microbiol* 78 (4): 1140–1147. doi.org/10.1128/AEM.06983-11.

15. **helped reduce abdominal pain in people with IBS:** Drouault-Holowacz S, Bieuvelet S, Burckel A, Cazaubiel M, Dray X, Marteau P. (2008). A double blind randomized controlled trial of a probiotic combination in 100 patients with irritable bowel syndrome. *Gastroenterol Clin Biol* 32 (2): 147–152. doi:10.1016/j.gcb.2007.06.001.

16. **can help slow things down and help your gut to heal:** Czerucka D, Dahan S, Mograbi B, Rossi B, Rampal P. (2000). *Saccharomyces boulardii* preserves the barrier function and modulates the signal transduction pathway induced in enteropathogenic *Escherichia coli*-infected T84 cells. *Infect Immun* 68 (10): 5998–6004.

17. **It also has immune-modulating benefits:** Gaby AR. (2011). *Nutritional medicine* (Concord, NH: Perlberg).

18. **taking glutamine supplements helps maintain the integrity of the gut barrier and improve immune function:** Ghouzali I, Lemaitre C, Bahlouli W, et al. (2017). Targeting immunoproteasome and glutamine supplementation prevent intestinal hyperpermeability. *Biochem Biophys Acta* 1861 (1 Pt A): 3278–3288. doi:10.1016/j.bbagen.2016.08.010; Wang B, Wu Z, Ji Y, Sun K, Dai Z, Wu G. (2016). L-glutamine enhances tight junction integrity by activating CaMK kinase 2-AMP-activated protein kinase signaling in intestinal porcine epithelial cells. *J Nutr* 146 (3): 501–508. doi:10.3945/jn.115.224857.

19. **Digestive enzymes help maintain the intestinal wall to keep bad microbes out:** Viggiano D, Ianiro G, Vanella G, et al. (2015). Gut barrier in health and disease: focus on childhood. *Eur Rev Med Pharmacol Sci* 19 (6): 1077–1085.

20. **Fish oil has a large amount of omega-3 fatty acids:** Gaby AR. (2011). *Nutritional medicine* (Concord, NH: Perlberg).

21. **fish oil in combination with probiotics enhances the intestinal cell lining:** Mokkala K, Laitinen K, Röytiö H. (2016). *Bifidobacterium lactis* 420 and fish oil enhance intestinal epithelial integrity in Caco-2 cells. *Nutr Res* 36 (3): 246–252. doi:10.1016/j.nutres.2015.11.014.

22. **Other studies have found similar results:** Zhao J, Shi P, Sun Y, et al. (2015). DHA protects against experimental colitis in IL-10-deficient mice associated with the modulation of intestinal epithelial barrier function. *Br J Nutr* 114 (2): 181–188.

23. **Krill oil is effective at lowering inflammation and protecting the gut wall:** Costanzo M, Cesi V, Prete E, et al. (2016). Krill oil reduces intestinal inflammation by improving epithelial integrity and impairing adherent-invasive *Escherichia coli* pathogenicity. *Dig Liver Dis* 48(1): 34–42. doi:10.1016/j.dld.2015.09.012.

24. **studies show that it is also useful in repairing leaky gut:** De Quelen F, Chevalier J, Rolli-Derkinderen M, Mourot J, Neunlist M, Boudry G. (2011). n–3 polyunsaturated fatty acids in the maternal diet modify the postnatal development of nervous regulation of intestinal permeability in piglets. *J Physiol* 589 (Pt 17): 4341–4352. doi.org/10.1113/jphysi.201011.214056.

25. **These help reduce inflammation, protect against heart disease and cancer:** Gambini J, Inglés M, Olaso G, et al. (2015). Properties of resveratrol: in vitro and in vivo studies about metabolism, bioavailability, and biological effects in animal models and humans. *Oxid Med Cell Longev* 2015: 837042. doi.org/10.1155/2015/837042.

26. **Resveratrol can stop gut inflammation and protect the intestinal barrier:** Bereswill S, Muñoz M, Fischer A, et al. (2010). Anti-inflammatory effects of resveratrol, curcumin and simvastatin in acute small intestinal inflammation. *PLoS ONE* 5 (12): e15099. doi.org/10.1371/journal.pone.0015099.

27. **It can mildly stop the Lyme organism from reproducing:** Goc A, Rath M. (2016). The anti-borreliae efficacy of phytochemicals and micronutrients: an update. *Ther Adv Infect Dis* 3 (3–4): 75–82. doi.org/10.1177/2049936116655502.

28. **It has also been shown to help with several neurological diseases, such as Alzheimer's and Parkinson's disease:** Malhotra A, Bath S, Elbarbry F. (2015). An organ system approach to explore the antioxidative, anti-inflammatory, and cytoprotective actions of resveratrol. *Oxid Med Cell Longev* 2015: 803971. doi.org /10.1155/2015/803971.

CHAPTER 4: THE LYME SOLUTION IMMUNE-BOOSTING DIET

1. **alterations in gut pH can affect the gut flora's production of short-chain fatty acids:** Den Besten G, van Eunen K, Groen AK, Venema K, Reijngoud D-J, Bakker

BM. (2013). The role of short-chain fatty acids in the interplay between diet, gut microbiota, and host energy metabolism. *J Lipid Res* 54 (9): 2325–2340. doi.org /10.1194/jlr.R036012.

2. **The acid environment in the natural world also affects the mineral content of foods:** Riebeek H. (2011). The Carbon Cycle. earthobservatory.nasa.gov/Features /CarbonCycle/printall.php.

3. **a more-alkaline diet can help reverse this ongoing acidification:** Schwalfenberg GK. (2012). The alkaline diet: is there evidence that an alkaline pH diet benefits health? *J Environ Public Health* 2012: 727630. doi.org/10.1155/2012/727630.

4. **vitamin D, which boosts the immune system:** Wimalawansa SJ. (2016). Nonmusculoskeletal benefits of vitamin D. *J Steroid Biochem Mol Biol* pii: S0960– 0760(16)30252-7. doi:10.1016/j.jsbmb.2016.09.016.

5. **Improves the health of bones and teeth and regulates genes that help prevent cancer development:** AlMatar M, AlMandeal H, Makky EA, et al. (2016). The physiological/pathophysiological significance of vitamin D in cancer, cardiovascular disorders and beyond. *Curr Drug Metab* (Dec 7); Ness RA, Miller DD, Li W. (2015). The role of vitamin D in cancer prevention. *Chin J Nat Med* 13 (7): 481– 497. doi:10.1016/S1875-5364(15)30043-1.

6. **Protect against neurological illness, including multiple sclerosis:** Schwalfenberg GK. (2012). The alkaline diet: is there evidence that an alkaline pH diet benefits health? *J Environ Public Health* 2012: 727630. doi.org/10.1155/2012 /727630.

CHAPTER 5: PREVENT AND TARGET ACTIVE INFECTION

1. **Its success at treating bacterial, yeast, and some parasite infections is well documented:** Li G, Ma X, Deng L, et al. (2015). Fresh garlic extract enhances the antimicrobial activities of antibiotics on resistant strains in vitro. *Jundishapur J Microbiol* 8 (5): e14814. doi.org/10.5812/jjm.14814.

2. **"odorless" garlic extracts, available from several companies, do not effectively kill microbes:** Ingels D. (1999). *The natural pharmacist: natural treatments for high cholesterol* (Roseville, CA: Prima Lifestyles).

3. **Allicin, an active ingredient in garlic, which is responsible for its strong odor, is highly effective at reducing the bacterial load for both Lyme disease and its co-infections:** Zhang Q, Zhang Y. (2006). Lyme disease and modern chinese medicine (New York: Sino-Med Research Institute).

4. **allicin and allitridi are extremely safe, with no known toxicity:** Mikaili P, Maadirad S, Moloudizargari M, Aghajanshakeri S, Sarahroodi S. (2013). Therapeutic uses and pharmacological properties of garlic, shallot, and their biologically active compounds. *Iranian J Basic Med Sci* 16 (10): 1031–1048.

5. **Artemisiae (*Artemisia annua*) capsules are widely used because of their efficacy in treating malaria:** Muangphrom P, Seki H, Fukushima EO, Muranaka T.

(2016). Artemisinin-based antimalarial research: application of biotechnology to the production of artemisinin, its mode of action, and the mechanism of resistance of *Plasmodium* parasites. *J Nat Med* 70: 318–334. doi.org/10.1007/s11418 -016-1008y.

6. **Artemisiae capsules have been shown to suppress the production of autoantibodies and reduce inflammatory molecules:** Yun C, Jung Y, Chun W, et al. (2016). Anti-inflammatory effects of *Artemisia* leaf extract in mice with contact dermatitis in vitro and in vivo. *Mediators Inflamm* 2016: 8027537. doi.org/10.1155/2016 /8027537; An J, Minie M, Sasaki T, Woodward JJ, Elkon KB. (2016). Antimalarial drugs as immune modulators: new mechanisms for old drugs. *Annu Rev Med* (Oct 21).

7. **enhances immune function by helping your tissues' immune cells more readily rid the body of bacteria and viruses:** Zhang Q, Zhang Y. (2006). Lyme disease and modern Chinese medicine (New York: Sino-Med Research Institute).

8. **as effective as some common antibiotics in stopping the growth of harmful bacteria:** Franzblau SG, Cross C. (1986). Comparative in vitro antimicrobial activity of Chinese medicinal herbs. *J Ethnopharmacol* 15 (3): 279–288.

9. **increasing white blood cell count, and enhancing immune activity:** Liu Y, Wang J, Wang W, Zhang H, Zhang X, Han C. (2015). The chemical constituents and pharmacological actions of *Cordyceps sinensis*. *Evid Based Complement Alternat Med* 2015: 575063. doi.org/10.1155/2015/575063.

10. **Cordyceps can also help reduce high blood pressure:** Yan XF, Zhang ZM, Yao HY, et al. (2013). Cardiovascular protection and antioxidant activity of the extracts from the mycelia of *Cordyceps sinensis* act partially via adenosine receptors. *Phytother Res* 27 (11): 1597–1604. doi:10.1002/ptr.4899.

11. **herbs in the formula supply additional antimicrobial activity, reduce inflammation, enhance detoxification, and help promote tissue repair:** Zhao Q, Chen X-Y, Martin C. (2016). *Scutellaria baicalensis*, the golden herb from the garden of Chinese medicinal plants. *Sci Bull* 61 (18): 1391–1398. doi.org/10.1007/s11434-016 -1136-5.

12. **particularly good for those experiencing brain fog or poor memory:** Carlson S, Peng N, Prasain JK, Wyss JM. (2008). The effects of botanical dietary supplements on cardiovascular, cognitive and metabolic function in males and females. *Gender Med* 5 (Suppl A), S76–S90. doi.org/10.1016/j.genm.2008.03.008.

13. **the combination of Samento and Banderol was effective at killing all three forms of *Borrelia burgdorferi* (the Lyme bacteria) in test-tube studies:** nutramedix.ec /pdfs/CAMResearch%20Article.pdf.

14. **killing biofilm-coated bacteria would require a higher-magnitude dose:** Haagensen JAJ, Verotta D, Huang L, Spormann A, Yang K. (2015). New in vitro model to study the effect of human simulated antibiotic concentrations on bacterial biofilms. *Antimicrob Agents Chemother* 59: 4074–4081.

15. **antibiotics may actually increase Lyme's biofilm production:** Sapi E, Kaur N, Anyanwu S, et al. (2011). Evaluation of in-vitro antibiotic susceptibility of different morphological forms of *Borrelia burgdorferi*. *Infect Drug Resist* 4: 97–113. doi.org /10.2147/IDR.S19201.

16. **vitamin D deficiency affects more than 40 percent of people:** Forrest KY, Stuhl-dreher WL. (2011). Prevalence and correlates of vitamin D deficiency in US adults. *Nutr Res* 31 (1): 48–54. doi:10.1016/j.nutres.2010.12.001.

17. **may affect up to two billion people worldwide:** Prasad AS. (2003). Zinc deficiency: has been known of for 40 years but ignored by global health organisations. *BMJ* 326 (7386): 409–410.

18. **doctors are finding it effective in treating rheumatoid arthritis and ulcerative colitis:** Jantan I, Ahmad W, Bukhari SN. (2015). Plant-derived immunomodula-tors: an insight on their preclinical evaluation and clinical trials. *Front Plant Sci* 6: 655. doi.org/10.3389/fpls.2015.00655.

CHAPTER 6: HIDDEN TOXINS IN YOUR SURROUNDINGS

1. **chemicals that have been associated with causing cancer, asthma, allergies, and other health issues:** Ye D, Klein M, Chang HH, et al. (2016). Estimating acute cardiorespiratory effects of ambient volatile organic compounds. *Epidemiology* (Dec 12); Kim J, Kim H, Lim D, Lee Y-K, Kim JH. (2016). Effects of indoor air pollut-ants on atopic dermatitis. *Int J Environ Res Public Health* 13 (12): 1220. doi.org /10.3390/ijerph13121220; St. Helen G, Jacob P, Peng M, Dempsey DA, Hammond SK, Benowitz NL. (2014). Intake of toxic and carcinogenic volatile organic com-pounds from secondhand smoke in motor vehicles. *Cancer Epidemiol Biomarkers Prev* 23 (12): 2774–2782. doi.org/10.1158/1055-9965.EPI-14-0548.

2. **making it more difficult to fight off infection:** Hosgood HD, Zhang L, Tang X, et al. (2011). Decreased numbers of CD4+ naïve and effector memory T cells, and CD8+ naïve T cells, are associated with trichloroethylene exposure. *Front Oncol* 1: 53. doi.org/10.3389/fonc.2011.00053; Vine MF, Stein L, Weigle K, et al. (2000). Effects on the immune system associated with living near a pesticide dump site. *Environ Health Perspect* 108 (12): 1113–1124.

3. **also disrupt the hormones and immune system:** Heindel JJ, Blumberg B, Cave M, et al. (2016). Metabolism disrupting chemicals and metabolic disorders. *Reprod Toxicol* pii: S0890–6238(16)30363-X. doi:10.1016/j.reprotox.2016.10.001; Kopras E, Potluri V, Bermudez ML, Williams K, Belcher S, Kasper S. (2014). Actions of endocrine-disrupting chemicals on stem/progenitor cells during development and disease. *Endocr Relat Cancer* 21 (2): T1–12. doi:10.1530/ERC-13-0360.

4. **The number of chemicals that can steadily accumulate in your body is strikingly high:** Rea W. (1994) *Chemical Sensitivity*, Vol. 2 (Boca Raton, FL: Lewis).

5. **the baby can be born with chronic immune problems, developmental delays, and an inability to process toxins on his or her own:** Ünüvar T, Büyükgebiz A. (2012).

Fetal and neonatal endocrine disruptors. *J Clin Res Pediatr Endocrinol* 4 (2): 51–60. doi.org/10.4274/Jcrpe.569.

6. **Persistent exposure to these chemicals can lead to:** niehs.nih.gov/research/supported/assets/docs/j_q/phthalates_the_everywhere_chemical_handout_508.pdf.

7. **only about 200 of them have ever been studied for their long-term safety:** cnn.com/2010/HEALTH/10/26/senate.toxic.america.hearing/.

8. **a compound called glyphosate, which the World Health Organization has recently stated likely causes cancer:** iarc.fr/en/media-centre/iarcnews/pdf/MonographVolume112.pdf.

9. **glyphosate may also alter immune function toward autoimmunity and create more inflammation:** Kumar S, Khodoun M, Kettleson EM, et al. (2014). Glyphosate-rich air samples induce IL–33, TSLP and generate IL–13 dependent airway inflammation. *Toxicology*, 325: 42–51. doi.org/10.1016/j.tox.2014.08.008.

10. **ingredients in Roundup are more than a thousand times as toxic as glyphosate:** gmoseralini.org/wp-content/uploads/2015/11/Seralini-career-JBPC_2015.pdf.

11. **they can cause a chronic inflammatory reaction that affects the brain:** sites.grenadine.co/sites/syncopate/en/aanp/items/231.

CHAPTER 7: MORE SLEEP, MORE EXERCISE, LESS STRESS

1. **If the circadian rhythm gets disrupted, it can lead to obesity, diabetes, depression, bipolar disorder, and seasonal affective disorder:** nigms.nih.gov/Education/Pages/Factsheet_CircadianRhythms.aspx.

2. **melatonin supplements are safe for children:** Goldman SE, Adkins KW, Calcutt MW, et al. (2014). Melatonin in children with autism spectrum disorders: endogenous and pharmacokinetic profiles in relation to sleep. *J Autism Dev Disord* 44 (10): 2525–2535. doi.org/10.1007/s10803-014-2123-9; Van Geijlswijk IM, van der Heijden KB, Egberts AC, Korzilius HP, Smits MG. (2010). Dose finding of melatonin for chronic idiopathic childhood sleep onset insomnia: an RCT. *Psychopharmacology* 212 (3): 379–391. doi.org/10.1007/s00213-010-1962-0.

3. **5-HTP also helps people with depression and anxiety:** Jacobsen JP, Krystal AD, Krishnan KR, Caron MG. (2016). Adjunctive 5-hydroxytryptophan slow-release for treatment-resistant depression: clinical and preclinical rationale. *Trends Pharmacol Sci* 37 (11): 933–944. doi:10.1016/j.tips.2016.09.001; Abdala-Valencia H, Berdnikovs S, McCary CA, et al. (2012). Inhibition of allergic inflammation by supplementation with 5-hydroxytryptophan. *Am J Physiol Lung Cell Mol Physiol* 303 (8): L642–L660. doi.org/10.1152/ajplung.00406.2011.

4. **contains a compound called theanine that calms anxiety and stress while helping you sleep:** White DJ, de Klerk S, Woods W, Gondalia S, Noonan C, Scholey AB. (2016). Anti-stress, behavioural and magnetoencephalography effects of an l-theanine-based nutrient drink: a randomised, double-blind, placebo-controlled, crossover trial. *Nutrients* 8 (1): 53. doi.org/10.3390/nu8010053.

5. **It also helps improve mood and concentration:** Camfield DA, Stough C, Farrimond J, Scholey AB. (2014). Acute effects of tea constituents L-theanine, caffeine, and epigallocatechin gallate on cognitive function and mood: a systematic review and meta-analysis. *Nutr Rev* 72 (8): 507–522. doi:10.1111/nure.12120.

6. **Relieve the effects of stress:** Kachan D, Olano H, Tannenbaum SL, et al. (2017). Prevalence of mindfulness practices in the US workforce: National Health Interview Survey. *Prev Chronic Dis* 14: E01. doi.org/10.5888/pcd14.160034.

7. **Reduce blood pressure and heart rate:** Shi L, Zhang D, Wang L, Zhuang J, Cook R, Chen L. (2016). Meditation and blood pressure: a meta-analysis of randomized clinical trials. *J Hypertens* (Dec 28). doi:10.1097/HJH.000000000000121.

8. **Reduce anxiety:** Gong H, Ni CX, Liu YZ, et al. (2016). Mindfulness meditation for insomnia: a meta-analysis of randomized controlled trials. *J Psychosom Res* 89: 1–6. doi:10.1016/j.jpsychores.2016.07.016.

9. **Promote better sleep:** Gong H, Ni CX, Liu YZ, et al. (2016). Mindfulness meditation for insomnia: a meta-analysis of randomized controlled trials. *J Psychosom Res* 89: 1–6. doi:10.1016/j.jpsychores.2016.07.016.

10. **Relieve pain:** Andersen TE, Vægter HB. (2016). A 13-weeks mindfulness based pain management program improves psychological distress in patients with chronic pain compared with waiting list controls. *Clin Pract Epidemiol Ment Health* 12: 49–58. doi.org/10.2174/1745017901612010049.

11. **a link between long-term EMF exposure and health risks:** who.int/peh-emf /about/WhatisEMF/en/index1.html.

12. **EMF exposure has been associated with certain types of cancer:** Belyaev I, Dean A, Eger H, et al. (2016). EUROPAEM EMF Guideline 2016 for the prevention, diagnosis and treatment of EMF-related health problems and illnesses. *Rev Environ Health* 31 (3): 363–397. doi:10.1515/reveh-2016–0011.

13. **Lyme disease tends to make your blood thick:** Platonov AE, Sarksyan DS, Karan LS, et al. (2015). [The blood coagulation system and microcirculatory disorders in ixodid tick-borne borreliosis caused by *Borrelia miyamotoi*]. *Ter Arkh* 87 (11): 26–32. [Article in Russian]

14. **Other benefits are improving mood and sleep:** Andrade FM, Pedrosa RP. (2016). The role of physical exercise in obstructive sleep apnea. *J Bras Pneumol* 42 (6): 457–464. doi:10.1590/S1806–37562016000000156; Archer T, Ricci S, Massoni F, Ricci L, Rapp-Ricciardi M. (2016). Cognitive benefits of exercise intervention. *Clin Ter* 167 (6): e180–e185. doi:10.7417/CT.2016.1965.

CHAPTER 8: ADVANCED PROTOCOLS

1. **Underactive thyroid:** Jonklaas J, Bianco AC, Bauer AJ, et al. (2014). Guidelines for the treatment of hypothyroidism: prepared by the American Thyroid Association Task Force on Thyroid Hormone Replacement. *Thyroid* 24 (12): 1670–1751. doi .org/10.1089/thy.2014.0028.

2. **Poor sleep patterns:** Russell C, Wearden AJ, Fairclough G, Emsley RA, Kyle SD. (2016). Subjective but not actigraphy-defined sleep predicts next-day fatigue in chronic fatigue syndrome: a prospective daily diary study. *Sleep* 39 (4): 937–944. doi.org/10.5665/sleep.5658.

3. **Poor or inadequate nutrition:** Barker LA, Gout BS, Crowe TC. (2011). Hospital malnutrition: prevalence, identification and impact on patients and the healthcare system. *Int J Environ Res Public Health* 8 (2): 514–527. doi.org/10.3390/ijerph 8020514.

4. **Depression:** Slavich GM, Irwin MR. (2014). From stress to inflammation and major depressive disorder: a social signal transduction theory of depression. *Psychol Bull* 140 (3): 774–815. doi.org/10.1037/a0035302.

5. **Mitochondrial dysfunction:** Morris G, Berk M. (2015). The many roads to mitochondrial dysfunction in neuroimmune and neuropsychiatric disorders. *BMC Medicine* 13: 68. doi.org/10.1186/s129160-015-0310-y.

6. **Defects in mitochondria have been associated with almost every chronic illness:** Morris G, Berk M. (2015). The many roads to mitochondrial dysfunction in neuroimmune and neuropsychiatric disorders. *BMC Medicine* 13: 68. doi.org/10.1186 /s129160–150–310-y.

7. **Lyme disease can reduce the number of, as well as damage, your mitochondria:** Peacock BN, Gherezghiher TB, Hilario JD, Kellermann GH. (2015). New insights into Lyme disease. *Redox Biol* 5: 66–70. doi.org/10.1016/j.redox.2015.03.002.

8. **Heart disease:** Fotino AD, Thompson-Paul AM, Bazzano LA. (2013). Effect of coenzyme Q10 supplementation on heart failure: a meta-analysis. *Am J Clin Nutr* 97 (2): 268–275. doi.org/10.3945/ajcn.112.040741.

9. **High blood pressure:** Borghi C, Cicero AF. (2017). Nutraceuticals with a clinically detectable blood pressure-lowering effect: a review of available randomized clinical trials and their meta-analyses. *Br J Clin Pharmacol* 83 (1): 1631–1671. doi:10.1111/bcp.12902.

10. **Hyperthyroidism:** Suzuki H, Naitoh T, Kuniyoshi S, et al. (1984). Cardiac performance and coenzyme thyroid disorders. *Endocrinol Jpn* 31 (6): 755–761.

11. **Migraine headaches:** Shoeibi A, Olfati N, Soltani Sabi M, Salehi M, Mali S, Akbari Oryani M. (2017). Effectiveness of coenzyme Q10 in prophylactic treatment of migraine headache: an open-label, add-on, controlled trial. *Acta Neurol Belg* (Sep 26).

12. **Alzheimer's disease:** Dumont M, Kipiani K, Yu F, et al. (2011). Coenzyme Q10 decreases amyloid pathology and improves behavior in a transgenic mouse model of Alzheimer's disease. *J Alzheimers Dis* 27 (1): 211–223. doi.org/10.3233/JAD -2011-110209.

13. **Parkinson's disease:** Yoritaka A, Kawajiri S, Yamamoto Y, et al. (2015). Randomized, double-blind, placebo-controlled pilot trial of reduced coenzyme Q10 for Parkinson's disease. *Parkinsonism Relat Disord* 21 (8): 911–916. doi:10.1016/j.park reldis.2015.05.022.

14. **AIDS:** Folkers K, Langsjoen P, Nara Y, et al. (1988). Biochemical deficiencies of coenzyme Q10 in HIV-infection and exploratory treatment. *Biochem Biophys Res Commun* 153 (2): 888–896.

15. **Hearing loss:** Staffa P, Cambi J, Mezzedimi C, Passali D, Bellussi L. (2014). Activity of coenzyme Q (Q-Ter multicomposite) on recovery time in noise-induced hearing loss. *Noise Health* 16: 265–269.

16. **Ringing in the ears:** Khan M, Gross J, Haupt H, et al. (2007). A pilot clinical trial of the effects of coenzyme Q10 on chronic tinnitus aurium. *Otolaryngol Head Neck Surg* 136 (1): 72–77.

17. **statin medications lower CoQ10 levels:** Ingels D. (2000). *Natural treatments for high cholesterol* (Rocklin, CA: Prima).

18. **people with Lyme disease who had neurological symptoms, such as memory problems, mood changes, poor balance, and neuropathy, had lower blood levels of carnitine:** Kępka A, Pancewicz SA, Janas RM, Świerzbińska R. (2016). Serum carnitine concentration is decreased in patients with Lyme borreliosis. *Postepy Hig Med Dosw* 70: 180–185.

19. **acetyl-L-carnitine may provide other health benefits beyond just enhancing your energy:** Liu J, Head E, Kuratsune H, Cotman CW, Ames BN. (2004). Comparison of the effects of L-carnitine and acetyl-L-carnitine on carnitine levels, ambulatory activity, and oxidative stress biomarkers in the brain of old rats. *Ann N Y Acad Sci* 1033: 117–131.

20. **ALA can reduce blood sugar and prevent neuropathy in diabetics:** Mijnhout GS, Kollen BJ, Alkhalaf A, Kleefstra N, Bilo HJ. (2012). Alpha lipoic acid for symptomatic peripheral neuropathy in patients with diabetes: a meta-analysis of randomized controlled trials. *Int J Endocrinol* 2012: 456279. doi.org/10.1155/2012/456279.

21. **Good research shows that vitamin B6 boosts energy:** Sun M, Qian F, Shen W, et al. (2012). Mitochondrial nutrients stimulate performance and mitochondrial biogenesis in exhaustively exercised rats. *Scand J Med Sci Sports* 22 (6): 764–775. doi:10.1111/j.16000–838.2011.01314.x; Heap LC, Peters TJ, Wessely S. (1999). Vitamin B status in patients with chronic fatigue syndrome. *J Royal Soc Med* 92 (4): 183–185.

22. **Bernie Rimland, PhD, studied the effects of vitamin B6 and magnesium in autistic children:** Rimland B, Callaway E, Dreyfus P. (1974). The effect of high doses of vitamin B6 on autistic children: a double-blind crossover study. *Am J Psychiatry* 135 (4): 472–475.

23. **many children with autism have mitochondrial issues:** Fatemi SH, Aldinger KA, Ashwood P, et al. (2012). Consensus paper: pathological role of the cerebellum in autism. *Cerebellum (London, England)*, 11 (3): 777–807. doi.org/10.1007/s12311-012-0355-9.

24. **at least one study suggests pyridoxine is better absorbed:** Middleton HM 3rd. (1979). Intestinal absorption of pyridoxal-5'-phosphate: disappearance from perfused segments of rat jejunum in vivo. *J Nutr* 109 (6): 975–981.

25. **PC has been used to treat many conditions:** Narayanan S, Nieh AH, Kenwood BM, et al. (2016). Distinct roles for intracellular and extracellular lipids in hepatitis C virus infection. *PLoS ONE* 11 (6): e0156996. doi.org/10.1371/journal .pone.0156996; Karner M, Kocjan A, Stein J, et al. (2014). First multicenter study of modified release phosphatidylcholine "LT-02" in ulcerative colitis: a randomized, placebo-controlled trial in mesalazine-refractory courses. *Am J Gastroenterol* 109 (7): 1041–1051. doi.org/10.1038/ajg.2014.104; Qureshi NA, Al-Bedah AM. (2013). Mood disorders and complementary and alternative medicine: a literature review. *Neuropsychiatr Dis Treat* 9: 639–658. doi.org/10.2147/NDT.S43419; Little A, Levy R, Chuaqui-Kidd P, Hand D. (1985). A double-blind, placebo controlled trial of high-dose lecithin in Alzheimer's disease. *J Neurol Neurosurg Psychiatry* 48 (8): 736–742.

26. **exposure to that type of EMF may disrupt normal organ function:** who.int/peh -emf/publications/Complet_DEC_2007.pdf?ua=1.

27. **PEMF generates low-level frequencies that stimulate blood flow and tissue repair:** Hao C-N, Huang J-J, Shi Y-Q, et al. (2014). Pulsed electromagnetic field improves cardiac function in response to myocardial infarction. *Am J Transl Res* 6 (3): 281–290; Reid B, Zhao M. (2014). The electrical response to injury: molecular mechanisms and wound healing. *Adv Wound Care* 3 (2): 184–201. doi.org/10.1089 /wound.2013.0442.

28. **European doctors have used PEMF to help heal broken bones:** Wang Q, Wu W, Han X, et al. (2014). Osteogenic differentiation of amniotic epithelial cells: synergism of pulsed electromagnetic field and biochemical stimuli. *BMC Musculoskelet Disord* 15: 271. doi.org/10.1186/1471-2474-15-271.

29. **PEMF has come into use in the United States for pain, stress, anxiety, and depression:** Thomas AW, Graham K, Prato FS, et al. (2007). A randomized, double-blind, placebo-controlled clinical trial using a low-frequency magnetic field in the treatment of musculoskeletal chronic pain. *Pain Res Manag* 12 (4): 249–258; Bech P, Gefke M, Lunde M, Lauritzen L, Martiny K. (2011). The pharmacopsychometric triangle to illustrate the effectiveness of T-PEMF concomitant with antidepressants in treatment resistant patients: a double-blind, randomised, sham-controlled trial revisited with focus on the patient-reported outcomes. *Depress Res Treat* 2011: 806298. doi.org/10.1155/2011/806298; Schoutens AM, Frings-Dresen MH, Sluiter JK. (2016). Design of a randomized controlled trial on the effect on return to work with coaching plus light therapy and pulsed electromagnetic field therapy for workers with work-related chronic stress. *BMC Public Health* 16: 597. doi.org /10.1186/s12889-016-3276-6.

30. **The risk of developing a life-threatening reaction during an allergy shot:** Lieberman P. (2012). The risk and management of anaphylaxis in the setting of immunotherapy. *Am J Rhinol Allergy* 26 (6), 469–474. doi.org/10.2500/ajra.2012 .26.3811.

31. **Although sublingual immunotherapy (SLIT) is not well known in the United States:** Fitzhugh DJ, Lockey RF. (2011). Allergen immunotherapy: a history of the first 100 years. *Curr Opin Allergy Clin Immunol* 11 (6): 554–559. doi:10.1097 /ACI.0b013e32834c3134.

32. **Sublingual immunotherapy has been researched extensively:** Canonica GW, Cox L, Pawankar R, et al. (2014). Sublingual immunotherapy: World Allergy Organization position paper 2013 update. *World Allergy Org J* 7 (1): 6. doi.org/10.1186 /1939-4551-7-6; Penagos M, Compalati E, Tarantini F, et al. (2009). Efficacy of sublingual immunotherapy in the treatment of allergic rhinitis in pediatric patients 3 to 18 years of age: a meta-analysis of randomized, placebo-controlled, double-blind trials. *Ann Allergy Asthma Immunol* 97 (2): 141–148; Wilson DR, Torres Lima M, Durham SR. (2005). Sublingual immunotherapy for allergic rhinitis: systematic review and meta-analysis. *Allergy* 60: 4–12. doi:10.1111/j.1398-9995.2005.00699.x; Compalati E, Passalacqua G, Bonini M, Canonica GW. (2009). The efficacy of sublingual immunotherapy for house dust mites respiratory allergy: results of a GA2LEN meta-analysis. *Allergy* 64 (11): 1570–1579. doi:10.1111/j.1398-9995 .2009.02129.x.

33. **In many countries throughout Europe, it is the preferred method:** Linkov G, Toskala E. (2014). Sublingual immunotherapy: what we can learn from the European experience. *Curr Opin Otolaryngol Head Neck Surg* 22 (3): 208–210. doi:10.1097 /M.000000000000000042.

34. **He and his group have since published several papers on the effectiveness of SLIT:** Morris MS, Lowery A, Theodoropoulos DS, Duquette RD, Morris DL. (2012). Quality of life improvement with sublingual immunotherapy: a prospective study of efficacy. *J Allergy* 2012: 253879. doi.org/10.1155/2012/253879; Theodoropoulos DS, Morris MS, Morris DL. (2009). Emerging concepts of sublingual immunotherapy for allergy. *Drugs Today* 45 (10): 737–750. doi:1396674/dot.2009 .45.10.1414893.

35. **Over ninety published studies document the efficacy of low-dose naltrexone (LDN) for various illnesses:** Mischoulon D, Hylek L, Yeung AS, et al. (2017). Randomized, proof-of-concept trial of low dose naltrexone for patients with break-through symptoms of major depressive disorder on antidepressants. *J Affect Disord* 208: 61–64. doi:10.1016/j.jad.2016.08.029; Tawfik DI, Osman AS, Tolba HM, Khattab A, Abdel-Salam LO, Kamel MM. (2016). Evaluation of therapeutic effect of low dose naltrexone in experimentally-induced Crohn's disease in rats. *Neuropeptides* 59: 394–395. doi:10.1016/j.npep.2016.06.003; Gironi M, Martinelli-Boneschi F, Sacerdote P, et al. (2008). A pilot trial of low-dose naltrexone in primary progressive multiple sclerosis. *Mult Scler* 14 (8): 1076–1083. doi:10.1177

/1352458508095828; Zagon IS, Rahn KA, Turel AP, McLaughlin PJ. (2009). Endogenous opioids regulate expression of experimental autoimmune encephalomyelitis: a new paradigm for the treatment of multiple sclerosis. *Exp Biol Med* 234 (11): 1383–1392. doi:10.3181/0906-RM-189; Liu WM, Scott KA, Dennis JL, Kaminska E, Levett AJ, Dalgleish AG. (2016). Naltrexone at low doses upregulates a unique gene expression not seen with normal doses: Implications for its use in cancer therapy. *Int J Oncol* 49 (2): 793–812. doi:10.3892/ij.20016.3567.

CHAPTER 9: AM I BETTER? HOW TO CYCLE BACK THROUGH THE FIVE-STAGE PLAN IF YOU'RE NOT

1. **Research shows that patients with early Lyme disease have high levels of proinflammatory cytokines:** Oosting M, Buffen K, van der Meer JW, Netea MG, Joosten LA. (2016). Innate immunity networks during infection with *Borrelia burgdorferi*. *Crit Rev Microbiol* 42 (2): 233–244. doi:10.3109/1040841X.2014.929563.

2. **patients with acute Lyme disease have elevated levels of C3a and C4a:** Stricker RB, Savely VR, Motanya NC, Giclas PC. (2009). Complement split products C3a and C4a in chronic Lyme disease. *Scand J Immunol* 69: 64–69.

3. **TGF-β1 increases in patients with early Lyme disease:** Widhe M, Grusell M, Ekerfelt C, Vrethem M, Forsberg P, Ernerudh J. (2002). Cytokines in Lyme borreliosis: lack of early tumour necrosis factor-α and transforming growth factor-β1 responses are associated with chronic neuroborreliosis. *Immunology* 107 (1): 46–55; Grygorczuk S, Chmielewski T, Zajkowska J, et al. (2007). Concentration of TGF-beta1 in the supernatant of peripheral blood mononuclear cells cultures from patients with early disseminated and chronic lyme borreliosis. *Adv Med Sci* 52: 174–178.

4. **Americans are surprised to learn that malnutrition and poor absorption are so common:** unicef.org/sowc98/feat03.htm.

5. **According to the Vitamin D Council, 40 ng/mL is the minimum:** vitamindcouncil.org/i-tested-my-vitamin-d-level-what-do-my-results-mean/.

6. **Patients with early Lyme disease have high levels of proinflammatory cytokines:** Glickstein L, Moore B, Bledsoe T, Damle N, Sikand V, Steere AC. (2003). Inflammatory cytokine production predominates in early Lyme disease in patients with erythema migrans. *Infect Immun* 71 (10): 6051–6053.

7. **Doctors long believed that the small intestine was mostly sterile:** Thadepalli H, Lou MA, Bach VT, Matsui TK, Mandal AK. (1979). Microflora of the human small intestine. *Am J Surg* 138 (6): 845–850.

8. **the small intestine simply harbors different kinds of bacteria than those found in the large intestine:** Chu H, Fox M, Zheng X, et al. (2016). Small intestinal bacterial overgrowth in patients with irritable bowel syndrome: clinical characteristics, psychological factors, and peripheral cytokines. *Gastroenterol Res Pract* 2016: 3230859. doi.org/10.1155/2016/3230859.

9. **many scientists believe it's a common cause of IBS:** Chu H, Fox M, Zheng X, et al. (2016). Small intestinal bacterial overgrowth in patients with irritable bowel syndrome: clinical characteristics, psychological factors, and peripheral cytokines. *Gastroenterol Res Pract* 2016: 3230859. doi.org/10.1155/2016/3230859.

10. **more effective than rifaximin at eradicating SIBO:** Chedid V, Dhalla S, Clarke JO, et al. (2014). Herbal therapy is equivalent to rifaximin for the treatment of small intestinal bacterial overgrowth. *Glob Adv Health Med* 3 (3): 16–24.

11. **Lyme disease can stimulate mast cells:** Talkington J, Nickell SP. (1999). *Borrelia burgdorferi* spirochetes induce mast cell activation and cytokine release. *Infect Immun* 67 (3): 1107–1115.

12. **Someone with MCAS will show elevated measures of these mast cell contents:** Molderings GJ, Brettner S, Homann J, Afrin LB. (2011). Mast cell activation disease: a concise practical guide for diagnostic workup and therapeutic options. *J Hematol Oncol* 4: 10.

13. **Quercetin has been shown to be more effective than some prescription medications:** Weng Z, Zhang B, Asadi S, et al. (2012). Quercetin is more effective than cromolyn in blocking human mast cell cytokine release and inhibits contact dermatitis and photosensitivity in humans. *PLoS ONE* 7 (3): e33805.

14. **The first-line medical treatment of MCAS is over-the-counter antihistamines:** Molderings GJ, Haenisch B, Brettner S, et al. (2016). Pharmacological treatment options for mast cell activation disease. *Naunyn-Schmiedebergs Arch Pharmacol* 389, 671–694.

15. **Cromolyn sodium, one of the most commonly used:** Cardet JC, Akin C, Lee MJ. (2013). Mastocytosis: update on pharmacotherapy and future directions. *Expert Opin Pharmacother* 14 (15): 2033–2045.

16. **people with chronic Lyme disease who have previously been treated with antibiotics have developed POTS:** Kanjwal K, Karabin B, Kanjwal Y, Grubb BP. (2011). Postural orthostatic tachycardia syndrome following Lyme disease. *Cardiol J* 18 (1): 63–66.

17. **If you do not exercise at all, then you may make this condition worse:** Mathias CJ, Low DA, Iodice V, Owens AP, Kirbis M, Grahame R. (2012). Postural tachycardia syndrome—current experience and concepts. *Nat Rev Neurol* 8 (1): 22–34.

18. **Several medications can also be used to treat POTS:** Garland EM, Celedonio JE, Raj SR. (2015). Postural tachycardia syndrome: beyond orthostatic intolerance. *Curr Neurol Neurosci Rep* 15 (9): 60.

APPENDIX A: LYME AND CO-INFECTIONS

1. **complications—which can even be fatal—with *Babesia*:** Vannier E, Gewurz BE, Krause PJ. (2008). Human babesiosis. *Infect Dis Clin North Am* 22 (3): 469–ix. doi.org/10.1016/j.idc.2008.03.010.

APPENDIX B: CURRENT CDC GUIDELINES FOR
THE TREATMENT OF LYME DISEASE

1. **current guidelines in the United States:** Wormser GP, Dattwyler RJ, Shapiro ED, et al. (2006). The clinical assessment, treatment, and prevention of Lyme disease, human granulocytic anaplasmosis, and babesiosis: clinical practice guidelines by the Infectious Diseases Society of America. *Clin Infect Dis* 43 (9): 1089–1134.

Index